Art Activities for Groups

Art Activities for Groups

Providing Therapy, Fun, and Function

Diane Fausek-Steinbach

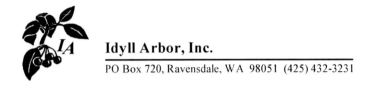

Idyll Arbor, Inc.

PO Box 720, Ravensdale, WA 98051 (425) 432-3231

Idyll Arbor, Inc. Editor: Thomas M. Blaschko

To the best of our knowledge, the information and recommendations of this book reflect currently accepted practice. Nevertheless, they cannot be considered absolute and universal. Recommendations for a particular client must be considered in light of the client's needs and condition. The author and publisher disclaim responsibility for any adverse effects resulting directly or indirectly from the suggested practices, from any undetected errors, or from the reader's misunderstanding of the text.

Library of Congress Cataloging-in-Publication Data

Fausek-Steinbach, Diane, 1963-

 Art activities for groups : providing therapy, fun, and function /
Diane Fausek-Steinbach.

   P. cm.

Includes bibliographical references and index.

 ISBN 1-882883-48-9

 1. Arts--Therapeutic use. I. Title.

 RC489.A72 F38 2002

 615.8'5156--dc21

             2002005343

ISBN 1-882883-48-9

Special thanks go to the editors and publishers of

Creative Forecasting Inc.

This book is dedicated to my most cherished husband, Norman.

You have made all my dreams come true.

Contents

Chapter One

Introduction

Benefits of Art as an Activity

The use of art processes as part of a group is beneficial for many reasons. It presents all populations with challenges in both the physical realm and the psychological realm. It allows the participant to internalize a concept, apply it to his or her own unique self, and to create a concrete expression of that process. This system of thought applies to all of your clients, from lowest to highest functioning, and even to you, yourself. Some of the basic goals and benefits of art as therapy are as follows:

Physical: Fine and gross motor skills are challenged. Clients with physical disabilities, paralysis, joint limitations, or shakiness due to disease process are challenged to complete a task with or without assistance. They may be asked to stretch farther, to use adaptive equipment to overcome, or to embrace their shaky lines as part of their own "style."

Clients with higher-level physical functioning may be challenged differently in regards to motor skills. They may be asked to assist another, or to work as part of a group, stretching to blend a mural,

1

manipulating a thin thread around a tree limb, or by using their own bodies as part of a living artwork.

Psychological: For clients with cognitive impairments, tasks involving color identification, following directions, and reminiscence are a challenge. The group leader may learn valuable information about the clients during a simple collage process that s/he may be able to share with other service providers, such as gauging levels of confusion and suggesting ways to reinforce reality orientation.

For a general population, a client is asked to self-evaluate, reflect on personality traits, goals, negative behaviors, and relationships. Art activities provide an opportunity to look at ourselves, and to see a self-portrait in many different forms: fabric collage, abstract watercolor paintings, anything we touch with a pencil or paintbrush.

The pairing of artist and art media, which is anything used in the process of creating, e.g., paint, clay, paper, nature objects, etc., is a very satisfying venture. The physical act of making art is therapeutic in and of itself. The irregular rhythm of paintbrush to paint, paint to canvas can hypnotize us, allowing us to put aside the internal dialogue we hear daylong and to lose ourselves in the creative process. The act of wedging clay, the systematic thud of clay on a board, kneading it back and forth as you would bread dough, can release stress and anxiety. Finger painting to music, feeling the wet, cool paint on the smooth surface while following a melody all leads us down a road of relaxation and timelessness.

As a therapist or activity leader, you are often faced with less than supportive comments about art programs and the resulting artwork. Remember that in art, as in life, it is the journey, not the destination, that brings us the most wealth.

Finding Your Inspiration

Creating meaningful and unique art experiences for your clients is a challenging and time consuming job, however, joining art media to issues of your population is really easier than you think.

Artists, art teachers, and art therapists are all offered a wide array of products to boost individual creativity. A stroll through your nearby fine arts supply or craft store may inspire many thoughts about how today's products can assist you in addressing your clients' needs. Products such as blank puzzles, blank playing cards, and blank rulers are some of the new products used in a few of the processes in this book. Using some of these products excites the artist because it offers new opportunity for theme related art imaging. It breaks the artist out of the mold of "draw or paint" and challenges ideas about what self-expression can be.

Traditional art media cannot be overlooked either! They, by their very nature of fluidity, texture, and color, can be used to inspire your clients to express themselves.

A trip through your supply cabinet or a flip through the pages of an art supply catalog is a great place to come up with inspiration.

How to Connect Media to Artists

In order to best help your clients successfully use art materials, you must look both at the nature of the materials and the nature of the artist. Find out what the artists' issues are and pair them with a medium that will either challenge them or let them feel safe, whichever is appropriate. For example, watercolor paints by their nature are fluid, unpredictable, colorfully intense, or obscure. They are hard to control for some, and require fast application.

How does that relate to your population? If your clients are confused, frightened by change, and have control issues, watercolor paints may be frustrating to them. They would be faced with the difficulty of trying to control something uncontrollable. If you want to challenge their abilities to "let go" and be spontaneous, perhaps an abstract watercolor-to-music process would be appropriate. If you want to focus on their issues of control and offer them a safe haven from a changing world around them, watercolors would not be a good medium.

Familiarity is also a good place to begin a challenge to your clients. Take a familiar object, story, or material, and add a twist. "The Cards You Are Dealt" process begins with a familiar object — a deck of cards — and then challenges the artist to put his/her own creativity to the test. Since the materials are familiar and easy to handle and manipulate, the artist is free to spend his/her time thinking and creating, instead of worrying about the unpredictability of the next 45 minutes.

Here is a general guide to media and client connections:

Medium/Nature	Client issues
Watercolor paints Fluid, unpredictable, hard to control, fast moving	High-level clients with control issues to challenge, low-level clients for sensory stimulation
Fabrics Familiar, textural, patterned	Great for the client who is confused, very recognizable and easy to relate to. Must be precut or prepared
Drawing pastels *Chalks* — can get intense colors on dark backgrounds, smudgy — good for blending colors or creating abstract art *Oil Pastels* — vibrant colors, easier application, creamy oil texture for blending, more of a fine-arts feel	Do not use with clients who are perfectionists and easily discouraged. The smudging can be very frustrating for some. Good to use with all high-level clients due to its ease of use and the fine quality results. Low-level clients may find it takes too much time to cover areas with color.
Clay — handbuilding Cold, stiff, must be handled with some knowledge of the medium, may have product loss through breakage in kiln, cracking as it dries	High-level clients who may not be spontaneous and like to be precise in the making of an art form. Must spend ample time teaching and learning the basics of clay work

Thinking "Adaptations"

When preparing a lesson plan for your group, think about the individuals and any special needs they may have. Always make sure that everyone in the group can do the process and create adaptations or adaptive equipment if needed.

For members of the group who have the use of only one hand or have problems with materials moving on them while they work, make small weight bags using sand or metal washers, covered in fabric. Think about raising the table with blocks of wood with a groove cut for the table leg for people in wheelchairs or Geri chairs. Precut materials if using scissors is difficult for your clients, making sure to offer enough variety of sizes and shapes. Try out your process before group time, look for possible frustrations, and come up with solutions before your clients have problems. Being quick with a fix alleviates the nervousness one might feel due to needing special help. When you have a complicated process in mind, recruit some volunteers or students to help each member along the way.

Getting Materials for Free

Art departments tend to get a variety of items donated by concerned and helpful family members and staff. Now I will tell you how to get the things you *want* for free! For fabrics, patterned and otherwise, develop a relationship with your local interior design or upholstery store. Go there in person, introduce yourself, explain a little about what you do and who you work for, and ask for any outdated sample books or end of bolt remnants they might have. Leave your name and number for them to call you when they have some for you to pick up and never turn it down no matter how much you may have accumulated. Share your wealth with art departments in other institutions. Art supply stores are sometimes willing to part with slightly damaged matte boards or papers, and again, meeting your new contact personally makes all the difference. If they can put a face, a name, and a good cause together you will indeed benefit from their generosity. Mention your ability to give them a public thank you with your displayed artwork. Your family members and staff are all possible customers for this business and will more likely go to a business they recognize as being a caring neighbor.

Using this Book with Clients

Finally, you are ready to proceed into a collection of tried and true art processes. Each process explains what population it may be best for, and any materials and adaptations needed. Read through the whole process before bringing it to your group to make sure it is appropriate for the member's "nature." Art is a powerful tool and should not be taken lightly. You are providing the opportunity for your clients to delve into their own psyche, to question and challenge themselves, and to stimulate thought about themselves and their environment. Make sure you allow them time to process their work and to discuss their feelings. Above all, know your group members, be prepared for any challenges they may throw at you, and allow for success and failure. The road to self-discovery is always filled with potholes.

Using this Book for Yourself

The plans in this book are good for your clients and you! Therapists, group leaders, and activity professionals are caregivers. We give of ourselves, we empathize with our clients, we get frustrated, we get tired, and we need nourishment for our souls and our spirits. When planning these sessions, I usually tried the process out on some colleagues and myself. It is nice to think about yourself for 20 minutes and talk to friends about what drives, motivates, and lives in our hearts. Self-examination is a valuable expenditure of time, as it can help us pinpoint why certain clients "trip our triggers," and why our hearts break sometimes when we see our clients struggle. Knowledge is power.

Try some of these processes out on yourself. Learn from the different media types, and the different challenges from each. Find out what relaxes you and what makes you feel confident.

Many of the following techniques are appropriate as team building "games" with your department or company. Using art among professionals as a team building method is a great way to identify common goals, fears, and strengths. The resulting artwork will only be as revealing as you want it to be. Your coworkers don't need to know all your hidden thoughts, but it is sometimes helpful to know the other members of your team on a more personal basis. We all need people around us that we can trust, and vent our frustrations and share our triumphs with.

How the Activities are Described

Each of the following art processes describes materials, clients, and the step-by-step path through the session. At the beginning of each new process, you will see a box of information to help you determine if that particular activity is appropriate for your group.

Size refers to the ideal number of clients in the group. This may vary with your individual circumstances. For example, if you have volunteers or students to assist you or if participants need direct hand over hand assistance, you may consider a different number of people for the group.

Functioning gives you a guide as to what cognitive and physical functioning levels your clients need in order to benefit the most from this specific process. This is not meant to be any kind of label, but needs to be mentioned in order to best match the process to the population.

Low level functioning would refer to clients who may be significantly cognitively impaired and disoriented, and who may also have some physical challenges as well, such as limited range of motion or visual difficulties.

Medium level would be a client with mild cognitive impairments who is able to stay on task with minimal reorientation and redirection. Physical limitations are overcome independently or with some assistance. For example, a person who has had a stroke, is somewhat forgetful, and has one-sided paralysis, but is able to converse or create in a determined way would fit into this category. I had a lady with Alzheimer's in my group for eight years. Her dementia progressed as we went along, but she was always ready to be creative and to continue to work on personal issues of loss, grief, and institutionalism. You can't tell about people by their diagnoses, so take time to get to know them before putting them into a group.

High level would refer to a person with minimal to zero physical or cognitive deterioration. These processes are meant to challenge one's self to the highest degree, to look at one's self and one's life with the goal of better self-understanding.

Time refers to the amount of actual group time a process takes. I believe in good preparation to insure a successful group, so having your materials ready and paints dispensed is important to the flow of the process.

Purpose relates to the goals, both psychological and physical of each process.

Chapter Two

Collages

A collage is the process of putting many pieces together to create a piece of art or object of self-expression.

Doing collages with your clients offers them a wide array of inspiration and possibilities. For low-level individuals, collage materials offer stimulation of most of their senses. Touch can be stimulated by feeling the differences in fabrics used in a project, or colors and feels of different papers. I feel working with natural items like branches, seashells, rocks, sand, etc. draw out a person's memories and link each person to the next. Some things are universal among us, and surely, even a disagreeable person will soften when looking back upon time spent as a youth climbing trees.

Collage projects also offer hesitant or "artistically challenged" individuals the opportunity to create easily and without the fear of looking foolish among other creative people. It allows people to think about the process, and the expression of thought, without having to struggle with the mechanics. Using mixed media as part of a painting or drawing offers a chance to be creative in a number of ways, giving the more creative person a chance to be more specific in his/her image making, while still incorporating some easy ready-to-go artwork.

With most of the following projects, however, you will need to place some limitations on materials. Allowing choices during art making is good, but don't feel the need to place all of the contents of your supply drawer on the table. Some clients will use everything you offer, creating a cluttered image that is more about experiencing all the materials than about exploring the process. Too much material stimulation will only confuse clients with dementia or moderate cognitive deficits. They will begin to get irritable regarding the "mess" and be frustrated with the process, unable to focus on cues and directions from you.

As always, knowledge of your clients' deficits and desires is most important in the success of your group. Invite them to explore materials and soon they will discover what they are most comfortable with, and what addresses their needs most effectively.

How to Collect Materials

Collecting and keeping collage materials is a double-edged sword. It is great to have what you need when you need it, but where, oh where, do you keep them?

It is imperative to have at least a moderate supply of collage materials available. Collect the worthwhile materials that lend themselves to many uses and discard the materials you always have been *taught* to use. In other words, throw away those egg crates and the 1000 copies of *National Geographic* that you have cluttering up your supply chest and make some room for the good stuff.

Have several types of fabrics handy. The sample books from interior design stores are great because they offer you a wide selection of colors and patterns all in one neatly bound book. Wallpaper samples come similarly bound and are a wonderful, *neat* way to organize your materials. Keep a bin of natural materials like twigs, stones, and shells. And a collection of, yes, magazines, but 12 copies should be all you need for a long time. Snippets of yarn and ribbons are not difficult to obtain from friends and families when you need them, so don't waste too much closet or storage space on that. Mostly, look at the world around you with an artist's eye and collect materials that awaken your senses and inspire you to create.

The Pile Up

Size	**3 to 8**
Functioning	**high (low or medium with modifications)**
Time	**40-60 minutes**
Purpose	**connectedness, group dynamics, abstract thinking, gross and fine motor skills**

Implementing group projects is always a challenge. Sometimes clients get so attached to their individual work they feel its effect is spoiled by being connected to the group. This process finds out if it is possible to be separate and together with others at the same time. Allowing the clients to have both personal pride in what they've done and to have pride in the fact that their own work can be part of something bigger is as important to personal development as creating individual artwork. The key to success is to find a connecting factor for the work, something that ties the pieces together.

The following process tackles this problem in a number of ways. First by supplying a common ground, by finding a theme, and by limited color choices. Second by layering the pieces in such a way that preserves each image's individuality. Unfortunately to do this you need to do some preparation work.

For this acrylic painting process the work surface is not paper but a matte board frame! You will have to cut (or buy) white matte frames in graduated sizes, each with a 3" border. So, for example, if you have 4 clients in your group, you need 4 surfaces: 3 frames in decreasing size and 1 centerpiece. It will look something like this.

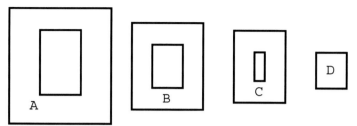

Fig. 2.1

For a group of 6 or 8, plan on separating the group in half with 3 or 4 pieces involved in each.

If you cannot get matte board, heavy poster board will also work, but it must be cut into a frame.

Materials

acrylic paints in blue, dark green, white, and deep red
paintbrushes and water buckets
soothing music, I use new age music, choosing a song that lasts about 20 minutes
Styrofoam or foam core spacers, 1" x 1" to put between layers of frames so that each frame sits on top of the one below it
hot glue, glue gun with hot glue sticks
palettes
trays

Preparation

1. Cut frames. Have paint dispensed into palettes, ready for distribution before group begins.

Activity

1. To begin the group, tell the participants that they will be working with color and music, but instead of working on paper, they will be painting on a matte frame piece that will later be put into a group image.

2.   Pass out frames. Determine your client's abilities and
            match the size of the frame to it. If Jane has limited
            range of motion, I will give her one of the smaller
            pieces. I will give the client who may need a self-esteem
            boost piece "A" (as it will be sitting on the top of the
            piece) if they are physically able to manipulate a frame
            that size. (Your biggest frame may be 24" x 28"!)

3.   Ask your clients to listen to selected music and to then
            paint how the music feels to them with the colors
            provided. Yes, they can mix colors.

4.   Allow 20 minutes to work.

5.   When all pieces are done, look at each piece
            individually. Can we tell if members of the group had
            the same response to the music by the color and
            movement of their frames?

6.   Next, beginning with the smallest piece, begin to lay the
            frames on top of each other. Place spacers in between the
            layers using the Styrofoam blocks to elevate and create a
            3-dimensional separation, like so:

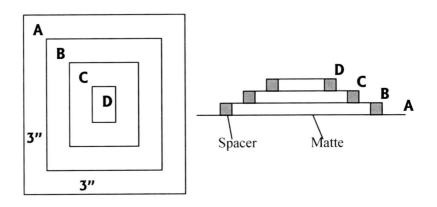

Fig 2.2

7.   Glue boards and spacers in place. Ask group members to evaluate the finished product. Do the individual pieces blend together and share common traits and feelings? Can they, as a group, decide on a title for the piece? With group projects like this, it is very important to let artists know that their individual work will be part of a group process. This prepares the client for the separation needed to put their work into place.

This group is especially satisfying in the sense that it takes individual abstract pieces and uses them to create a very visually exciting final piece. Somehow giving the abstract some concrete form. It can also be done with medium-level clients and clients that can follow one- or two-step directions. The goals for this group with high-level clients are increasing and challenging group dynamics, and abstract thinking development. With low-level clients your goals may be to increase abilities to follow one- or two-step directions, fine and gross motor skills, decision-making, and acknowledging others in the group.

Display the artwork along with the titles of the pieces.

Low Level Color Collage

Size	**1 to 6**
Functioning	**low**
Time	**20-40 minutes**
Purpose	**sensory stimulation, reminiscing, reality orientation**

Not every day is sunny and bright. Not every room or activity area is either! This collage is very stimulating, especially for clients with cognitive deficits or poor vision because they are working with and surrounded by color.

The following process uses bright transparent colors to stimulate reminiscence among clients with lower cognitive and physical functioning. This particular session was done in springtime, when gloomy, rainy days turn into sunny flower-filled gardens! You can use this theme or adapt it to fit your season or needs.

Materials

transparent cellophane in various colors
clear cellophane tape
scissors
white poster board, half sheet

Preparation

1.   Cut the transparent cellophane into large (hand size) geometric pieces.

Activity

1.   Lay white poster board in the middle of the table with 6 or fewer lower-level clients.

2.   Distribute some of the colored cellophane pieces on the table near the client's hands. Or, if balance is not a problem, encourage mild stretching by placing the colored cellophane pieces within reaching distance.

3.   Begin the group by talking about current weather condition, day, and date. Talk about spring approaching, and ask what kind of weather the participants like the best.

4.   Discuss the best part of spring as being the blooming of the flowers and all the beautiful colors that come out.

5.   Going to each participant, pick up a color of cellophane and ask the client to identify the color and shape of the piece.

6.   Ask: "Can you think of something else that is this color?" Suggest flowers or fruits that they could relate to.

7.   Ask the client to hold the shape and lay it somewhere on the white poster board. Tape the piece in place.

8.   Continue around the table in this manner. Invite the other participants to identify with the colors as a group. Tape pieces onto the board as you go, encourage overlapping, and then identify the new color!

9.   Continue to fill the board with shapes and colors. Invite the group to discuss colors by asking questions such as, "What is your favorite color? Do any of these colors match what you are wearing? What color are your eyes? What color is an apple?"

10.   When the board is completed, place it in the day room as a colorful reminder of your group, invite other staff to use the board as a sensory stimulation tool in the room during slow times, and instruct them in what questions to ask and how to stimulate discussion.

Options

- Cut the cellophane into shapes like flowers, fruits, or anything else the color relates to. Ask group members to apply the images onto the board, discussing each shape as they go.

- Use colored construction paper instead of cellophane for easier handling by lower-level clients.

- Apply cellophane to the sticky surface of clear contact paper. Once pieces are put on, sandwich them with another piece of clear contact and hang in a window as a "stained glass" sun catcher. Sheets can also be cut into flower or butterfly shapes for more decorative window art.

Magic Seeds

Size	**4 to 8**
Functioning	**medium to high**
Time	**40-60 minutes**
Purpose	**remotivation, reminiscing, fine motor control, sensory stimulation, abstract thinking**

The planting of a seed or tree is sometimes done as a response to a change in someone's life, as a living symbol of growth and nurturing of the future. We plant trees as memorials for loved ones, something that will exist long after our days have passed. We give seeds to new parents as a symbol of their joyful task to assist and teach a new soul to grow. If only we had magic seeds that would allow us to grow other things that we, as a community, as individuals, or as a universe need to grow healthy and productive. If you had magic seeds, what would you grow?

Materials

small terra cotta pots, enough for one per member of group
acrylic paints, brushes, water containers
soil
seeds (sunflower or marigold seeds work well)
ceramic gloss sealer spray

Activity

1. Begin the group with a discussion of nurturing. Ask: "How have we helped things to grow and develop through our lives? (Raising children, teaching values, loving others)"

2.   Ask: "What are some things that we wish we could give to others, to the community, or to the world to make it a better place? (Happiness, unconditional love, good health, good friends)"

3.   Imagine now that you have magic seeds so you have the ability to make that happen, to actually *grow* love, grow happiness, and grow laughter. Imagine that you have that ability.

4.   Distribute the empty terra cotta pots and paints. Ask the participants to think about what they would like to give the world and to paint an image of that on the outside of the pot. They can create an image of that feeling through symbols, colors, or words, however they want to express it.

5.   Allow 20 minutes to work.

6.   As the pots are being finished, take them outside and spray them lightly with the sealer. (Or do this project in two sessions. Make sure that you have a way to identify each person's pot by name or other identifying mark.)

7.   Next, have the clients fill their pots with soil and have them select seeds. Before they plant them, ask them to talk about what they hope to magically grow. Ask how it relates to the image on their pots.

8.   Finish the group with a discussion of nurturing and care giving. Ask: "How do we nurture those around us. Is there more we can do?"

Group members may take their plants back to their rooms, or grow them together in your day room or group room for all to enjoy.

Celebration

Size	4 to 12
Functioning	medium to high
Time	40-60 minutes
Purpose	self-worth, reminiscing, group bonding

Proposing a toast at a celebration or gathering of friends is a tradition in our culture. Weddings, anniversaries, or special meals are often blessed with a toast to good friends and good health. The feeling of celebration is often significantly lacking in the lives of clients who are in long-term care or other institutions, but, perhaps, with a change of perspective we can look at our daily lives and find many reasons to celebrate. This process uses (plastic) champagne glasses as both an art medium and a symbol for celebration among friends.

Materials

> plastic champagne glasses, 2 per client, (available at most party supply stores)
> tissue paper torn into small pieces
> confetti
> Modge Podge™ glue
> metallic paints
> small to medium size paintbrushes
> non-alcoholic champagne
> small sand bags to weigh down cups

Activity

1.   Begin with a discussion on the tradition of toasting. Can they remember proposing a toast? Perhaps at a holiday dinner or special gathering.

2.   Since most toasts are done with champagne, pass out the plastic champagne glasses (one per client) and instruct that they are to think of past celebrations and decorate their glasses as they desire, using the materials available. Modge Podge can be used to adhere the tissue paper and confetti if desired.

3.   Instruct your clients to decorate the outside of the glasses only.

4.   Turn glasses upside down to make decorating easier. Place a sandbag on the top of the glass or inside the glass to keep it from slipping and moving about.

5.   As they are finishing, ask them to share their finished glass with the rest of the group. Does it look festive? What memory were they thinking of as they worked?

6.   As the decorated glasses dry, pour champagne into the extra, unpainted glasses and distribute.

I take this opportunity to propose a toast to my group members for sharing their time and talents with me. I then invite other group members to make a toast if they desire.

All the members involved, both high and medium-level, enjoyed this process and the opportunity to "sit at the head of the table" again, to be the toastmaster, to celebrate together.

Patchwork Collage

Size	**2 to 6**
Functioning	**low, confused**
Time	**20-40 minutes**
Purpose	**sensory stimulation, pattern recognition, reminiscing, following one-step directions**

The following process is designed for use with clients with greater cognitive and/or physical difficulties. I use donated and elaborately designed wallpaper samples and one-step directions to complete this project. The goals: to visually interest and involve clients who are confused, to challenge abilities to follow directions, and to identify pattern and linear design. You will need wallpaper samples to complete this project. My suggestion to you would be to call local interior design establishments and request their donation of out of print or discontinued wallpaper sample books. If you are unable to find wallpaper, wrapping paper or solid colored paper will also do fine.

Since you will be working with clients with limited fine motor skills, you will need to do some preparation work ahead of time.

Materials

wallpaper samples (or wrapping paper or solid colored paper)
11" x 15" black construction paper to use as background paper to glue your strips onto
glue sticks

Preparation

1.   Cut the wallpaper samples into strips of various widths and linear design (e.g., wavy, straight, jagged), but all

15" long. Match the length of your strips to the length of the paper you choose to work with.

Activity

1.   Begin by laying black construction paper in front of clients.

2.   Next, scatter some of the wallpaper strips on the table. Encourage the clients to look through them. Ask: "Which colors do you like? What kind of pattern is that? Flowers? Lines? Is the paper fat or skinny? What does it feel like? (A lot of wallpaper samples are bumpy or slick.)"

3.   Ask them to choose some that they like, or place 2 or 3 strips in front of them.

4.   Ask them to lay the strip down on the paper. For example: "Pick up the pink paper. Lay it on the black paper, put it anywhere that you want." For clients who can only follow one-step directions, wait for then to pick up the paper before telling them what to do with it.

5.   Angle the strips on the paper in left to right linear placement as they pick and place strips.

6.   Glue down and continue.

You may find that many clients who are confused like orderliness and appreciate the "lining up" of the samples against the dark background. They may naturally try to organize by color or shape. The placement of the strips against the background helps separate the shapes and provides an opportunity for the eye to rest.

When you choose the samples to use, choose a variety of solids, floral, and other small patterns, watching for patterns and colors that may be recognized by your clients.

Although simple, this process offers many challenges to the cognitively impaired or confused individual, and creates a neat and exciting visual image they can refer or relate to.

Shadow Puppets

Size	**4 to 12**
Functioning	**medium to high (low with assistance)**
Time	**40-60 minutes**
Purpose	**reminiscing, play, creative expression, interactions with others**

Casting shadows and manipulating form have been pastimes for many a child. The time we spent perfecting that shadow puppet dog or bird in flight is pleasantly recalled during this process, which takes the familiar creation of shadow puppets of childhood and adapts it to the creative processes and often-restricted movement of the adult.

Materials

dowels, 1/4" diameter, at least 5" long
black construction paper
scissors
glue sticks
tape
light source (an overhead projector lamp is
recommended but a large bulb flashlight or slide
projector will also work fine)

Preparation

1.   Cut some shapes out of the black construction for those who cannot cut. Cut "parts," e.g., snout shapes, ears, and geometric shapes they can layer to create the look they desire.

Activity

1.   Plan group to be held in a room that can be darkened easily.

2.   Begin group with a discussion of shadow puppets. Ask: "Do you remember making shadow puppets on your bedroom walls as kids? What were some of the shapes you could make?"

3.   Explain that they will be taking the well-known shadow puppet to a different level by creating a shadow not with their hands, but with a form they create by cutting and pasting paper together.

4.   Distribute the black construction paper; scissors, glue sticks, and precut shapes. Ask them to assemble a form to cast a shadow. Their creation doesn't have to resemble an animal or anything reality based. They should only attempt to create an image with interesting silhouette possibilities.

5.   Assist with the gluing and cutting as necessary. Finished shapes should be no larger than 7" x 7" as the dowels can only support a shape of this size successfully.

6.   When the shapes are complete, tape a dowel to the back of the shape so that it can be held as a puppet.

7.   Ask participants if they would like to try out their puppets and inform them that you will need to darken the room.

8.   Turn on the light source, and darken the room. Allow each participant the opportunity to see his/her shape cast upon the wall. Encourage participants to allow their images to interact with other creations in a shadow play.

This group was originally designed for high to medium-level participants, but can be done also with medium to low-level clients with more assistance provided. Allow them to layer precut construction paper shapes into an image and tape to dowel. Even the lower-level participants may recall the shadow casting of the past and enjoy the reminiscence.

Medals of Honor

Size	**4 to 12**
Functioning	**medium (with help) to high**
Time	**40-60 minutes**
Purpose	**self-worth, self-expression, belonging to a group**

A "medal" is defined by Webster as: "a coin shaped piece of metal impressed with a device or inscription commemorating some distinguished event or person." It is a decoration, a prize, and an honor. Medals have been given to individuals over the centuries in recognition of achievement. Wouldn't it be nice to recognize the achievements we've made in our lives that may not have been noticed by anyone but ourselves? That is the basis for the following process that involves high to medium-level functioning clients in self-recognition, self-esteem building, and creativity.

Materials

fabric squares in a variety of patterns, colors, and textures to be cut into 2" x 5" or larger ribbons (be sure to have some metallic fabrics also!)
small gold safety pins
scissors
2" x 2" squares of black poster board
black permanent markers
glitter
glue (white and in stick form)
old jewelry
small needle nose pliers (to bend or clip off clasps or jewelry backings)
hot glue

examples of ribbons or award medals

Activity

1.   Have fabric laid out on table as group members enter the room.

2.   Begin a discussion about medals and awards. Ask: "Why do people receive them? What medals are you familiar with? (Olympic medals, Medals of Honor) Have you ever received a medal or recognition of some kind?"

3.   Discuss "medal's" definition and thoughts about receiving medals and ribbons for personal achievements. Ask: "What have you done that you deserve a medal for?" Give examples, such as being a good parent, being a good listener or friend, making people smile, persevering, etc.

4.   Next ask them to choose a fabric to make their ribbon from and assist with cutting it into desired ribbon length and width. (If someone wants a 4" wide ribbon, go ahead. Remember no rules!)

5.   Next, ask them to elaborate on their ribbon either by design or in words why the ribbon is being awarded. Cut other fabrics, glue, or provide markers as necessary.

6.   Now, place selected jewelry (pins and clip earrings work best) and squares of poster board out. Tell them that they can cut the poster board into any shape (star, oval, etc.) and hot glue a piece of jewelry to it if desired. They may also add glitter at this stage if they like. Glue the jewelry and poster board to the end of the ribbon.

7.   Attach the gold safety pin to the top of the ribbon when all the work on the medal is complete.

8.   When all participants are done, clear the table for the ceremonial pinning.

9.   At this point I go around to each member of the group, ask them what the medal is for, and with much pomp and circumstance present the participant with the medal and pin it on his/her shirt.

10.   The other group members applaud.

This group is done in a lighthearted manner, however it can be very revealing to the artist. If a group member cannot think of a reason s/he deserves a medal, the other group members make suggestions, or you may want to congratulate the person on progress in your group, in smiling more, or sharing more ideas with others. Everyone has earned a medal; some just have to understand why.

Strata Collage

Size	**2 to 6**
Functioning	**low to moderate**
Time	**20-40 minutes**
Purpose	**sensory stimulation, reminiscing, long-term memory, following one-step directions**

The following process is designed for clients who function at a low to medium cognitive functioning level. It explores color and shape and group interactions in a stimulating and aesthetically interesting way. Clients with memory deficits learn and remember things, if only briefly, by exercising their brains. Giving them the opportunity to identify color, shapes, and textures allows them to grasp a concept that goes back in their long-term memory and makes them feel successful in a world that they may often find frustrating and scary.

This process uses precut shapes and one-step directions to allow each participant to actively create in a non-threatening group process.

Materials

heavy construction paper in orange, pink, black, and green
poster board in blue, yellow, and red
glue sticks
scissors

Preparation

1. Cut a strip of poster board of each color approximately 10" wide and the length of the average sheet of poster board. Strips will look like this:

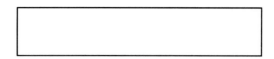

2.   Cut the following shapes out of the various colors of
            construction paper, about 5 of each, no larger than 10".

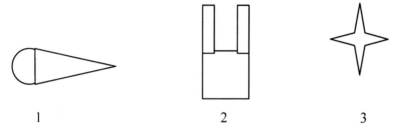

1   2   3

Activity

1.   Lay one sheet of poster board and 5 pieces of the same
            shape on the worktable.

2.   With the clients gathered around the table, take turns
            identifying the color of the pieces of construction paper.
            Look at the shape. Does it remind them of anything?
            Turn the shape in different directions. Does it resemble
            anything they can think of? For example, shape 1 may
            look like an ice cream cone; shape 2 may look like a
            dog, etc.

3.   Give each client one-step directions to:

            •   Take a colored shape.

            •   Lay it anywhere on the strip of poster board.

            Continue around table till that strip of poster board is
            filled. Overlapping is ok. Glue in place with the glue
            stick.

4.   Remove board, and replace it with a different color of
            poster board and a different set of shapes. Repeat the
            identifying and placing of shapes onto the poster board.

Repeat process with the third piece of poster board and the last set of shapes.

5.   When complete, Lay strips of poster board together to display. You should end up with something like this.

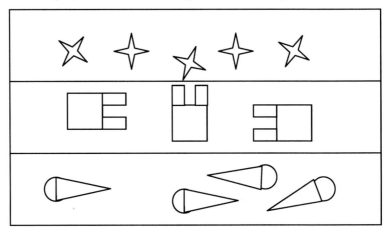

Experiment with different color and shape combinations for different looks. This process can be done with seasonal shapes as well, e.g., firecrackers, tulips. It can be theme related, e.g., *transportation* could include car shapes, trains, roller-skates, *tools* could include hammer shapes, saw blades, nuts and bolts, or even *babies*, which would include diaper shapes, baby bottles, teddy bears. Whatever you can think of that your clients may be able to both reminisce about and have the opportunity to identify the shapes and colors of, would be a stimulating and fun process. Hang the finished product in the day or community room to use with clients who have lower cognitive functioning as a one-on-one tool or for one-on-one sensory stimulation.

Links

Size	**6 to 10**
Functioning	**any level (low with assistance)**
Time	**30-60 minutes**
Purpose	**group membership, remotivation, abstract thinking**

What connects one person to another? Is it the bonds of blood, brother or sister? Is it the bonds of matrimony, husband and wife? Are people bound together by beliefs and dreams, by religion or creed? All of these things create a unity among people that is unseen but recognized. Being part of an art activity group creates a bond among artists and friends that is just as special, fragile, and important. The following process takes an unseen bond among group members and gives it color and movement.

Materials

poster board cut into strips 7" wide and 18" long, in
   different colors
craypas
metallic paints
white glue
glitter
fabric scraps
stapler

Activity

1.   Place strips of poster board on the table within participant's reach. Have enough of all colors for every individual to have his/her color choice.

2.   Begin group by discussing how things are connected. Ask: "How many different kinds of connections can you name?" (See introduction).

3.   Let them know that they will be creating "links." Using the materials provided they should create a representation of themselves. Ask them to use the colors and collage materials to create the "feel" of their personality, and of, perhaps, even their role as they see it within the group. For example, if I feel that I am the "clown" of the group, I may use bright colors and cheery images on my link. If I feel I am more somber, I may use more peaceful lines and dark colors.

4.   Allow 20 minutes for participants to create their links.

5.   When all are complete, ask each artist to describe his/her link and how it relates to self and to the group.

6.   Now make a first link by creating a circle with the poster board as you would to make a bracelet, and staple it shut.

7.   Next, ask for a second link and make the circle so that it is interlocked with the first, like a chain link, and continue the process.

8.   When all links are connected, hang the unit as a whole from the ceiling, from the top link so that the rest hang straight down.

9.   Ask the participants to comment on the final image. Ask: "What does this linkage say to us about connections among our group? Do the links create a stronger image together or separated?"

Display the links in your group room as a reminder of the importance of each member to the group. When new members are introduced to the group, ask them to create a link and add it to the image to solidify their belonging to the other members of the group.

Sharper Image

Size	**2 to 6**
Functioning	**low**
Time	**20-40 minutes**
Purpose	**motor skills, sensory stimulation, one-step directions, reality orientation**

The following group process is geared toward the lower level clients who may have difficulty with complex thoughts. It involves one-step directions (e.g., "Pick a blue piece.") and challenges the participants to be involved in a group art process. This group also provides opportunities for color association and motor skill tasks.

You will be using brightly colored construction paper and "action" shapes to capture the attention of the more confused clients and to create a dynamic image when complete. Asking the clients to connect the colored paper in their hands with the true colors of their environment is great for reality orientation and challenges the client to make associations between abstract and concrete. ("The paper is green, the grass is green, too.")

You could also do this project on a much larger scale, using a background piece of 28" or more and larger action shapes. This would be beneficial for those with significant visual deficits and is great for range of motion and gross motor skills.

Materials

precut construction paper shapes in miscellaneous bright colors
one full size (12" x 18") sheet of red construction paper
glue sticks
one sheet of black poster board

Preparation

1.   Cut various colors of construction paper into many sizes of sharp edged shapes like these:

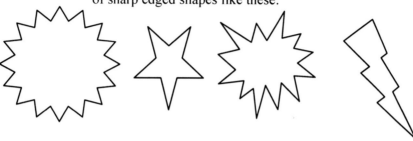

Fig 2.4

Activity

1.   Begin the group by talking about doing a collage using different shapes and colors of paper.

2.   Lay the large piece of red construction paper on the table. Ask clients to identify the color. Can they identify things that are the same color?

3.   Distribute one or two precut shapes to each group member. Ask them to identify the color and relate it to something else they know, e.g., "The paper is blue and so is my shirt."

4.   One at a time, ask them to place a shape on top of the paper. Assist with gluing in place if necessary, and continue the process until all of the participants have placed several pieces (as time allows).

5.   When all have placed and glued their shapes to the group's satisfaction, mount the entire piece on a black poster board. Display as a visual stimulation piece.

Since this group is geared for the lower cognitive level clients, its goals are met through increased motor skills, color identification, and awareness of others in a group environment.

Changing Reflections

Size	4 to 8
Functioning	**high**
Time	**40-60 minutes**
Purpose	**creativity, alternate viewpoints, reminiscing, self-image exploration**

Mirrors are part of our world. Through all our lives, they have told us how we look to others and ourselves. What if we could manipulate that image by manipulating the mirror itself? Much like the "funny mirrors" at the local fair midway, we can have fun with our image by layering small craft mirrors onto a sturdy flat background, and creating a mosaic of reflections, a kind of kaleidoscopic view of ourselves.

Materials

small craft mirrors approximately 1" to 3" in size, in square shapes or circles, generally available at most craft stores

heavy poster board or matte board 8" x 10"

hot glue or epoxy

foam core board or Styrofoam approximately 1/4" thick, cut into cubes (to be used as spacers.)

Activity

1. Begin discussion of "reflections." Ask: "What part of us does the mirror reflect? How we *feel* about ourselves is not visible in the reflection of a mirror." Discuss the use of mirrors in your project. Ask: "How have mirrors been used in our world as a design element? (in mosaics, on ornaments, kaleidoscopes, and even disco glitter balls!)"

2.   Distribute background matte or poster board and mirrors.

3.   Ask the group to create a design with their mirrors on the background piece. They should allow only small spaces between mirrors and try to use more than one shaped mirror.

4.   Assist with gluing these in place.

5.   Pass out Styrofoam or foam core spacers. Discuss how they can create dimension in their piece by "layering" some of the mirrors. Glue spacers on top of the mirror image already created and adhere another mirror piece to top of spacer, creating 3-dimensional images.

6.   After all of the pieces are glued in place, have clients look into their work. What does the layering of mirrors do to the image they see? How does that image change depending upon what is in front of it, or surrounding it?

This process not only allows the individual to creatively use a new medium in an art process, but also to get a view of themselves and their surroundings that is fun and has been completely manipulated by them. It is a great way to introduce your clients to multimedia projects and to experiment with the use of reflection devices in an art project.

Bits and Pieces

Size	**2 to 6**
Functioning	**low (higher with adaptations)**
Time	**20-60 minutes**
Purpose	**group interactions, self-worth, fine motor skills, color and pattern identification**

Bits and Pieces was created to encourage low level cognitive or physically functioning participants to interact with one another in a group forum, to stretch their abilities to accept the trespasses of others into their world, and to give them pride in the accomplishment of a group process. It can be utilized with higher level functioning clients successfully by upgrading materials and by allowing them to do more of the individualizing of the materials.

Materials

a variety of patterned or textured papers: wallpaper
samples or gift wrap are good, but for a higher "art"
look and for the more demanding higher functioning
artists, you may want to invest in some fine art
textured papers like Thai marbled or banana paper,
or fun papers like animal fur or flower patterns
available at your local fine art supply store
black poster board, 8" x 11" for higher level groups, 11"
x 17" for lower level
glue sticks

Preparation

1. For lower level group, cut or tear as many different
    shapes and patterns of paper as there are members of the

group. For example, it you have 6 group members, have 6 different patterns of paper, and have each different paper selection cut or torn into 1 of 6 different shapes. Have both very large and smaller pieces available. (No smaller than a quarter though, for ease of manipulation.)

2.   Higher level group, have as many different kinds of paper as there are people in the group.

Activity

3.   Have the one piece of black poster board laid out on the work surface in the middle of the group. This is your background piece.

4.   Discuss the meaning of "collage." Talk about creating a piece of artwork as a group, reflecting everyone's individual efforts.

5.   Ask each group member to select one style of paper that they are most attracted too. Ask the individuals why they chose that particular paper, Ask: "What about that paper did you like?" For lower level clients ask them to describe the pattern or texture of their paper. Ask them direct questions such as, "Is it rough or smooth, pink or blue?"

6.   Passing the black poster board around the table, ask each person to place one piece of paper on the board and glue it in place.

7.   Encourage people to use the entire surface of the board and to overlap and cross pieces as the board gets full. Rotate the board's direction occasionally to encourage spreading the materials out across the board.

8.   Continue to go around the table until the board has reached a satisfactory level of coverage, or is the most aesthetically pleasing. Let the group members decide

when to stop, and be prepared with another board in case they fill their board too quickly.

9.   When the piece is finished, look at it as a group. Trim off any overhanging pieces and make sure all of the pieces are glued securely.

10.   Ask the group to come up with a title for the piece.

Options

1.   You can offer the option of pooling left over scraps of paper from the first project and allowing group members to create smaller individual projects (5" x 7" boards).

Close the group discussion by talking about how it felt to combine forces to create one unified piece of art. Can they see themselves, their individually chosen or torn paper, in the mass? How did it feel to have to give up control? Can they see by the finished project that it was a struggle or that it was a cohesive experience?

As always, this type of project is great to begin new clients with, or to get all of those hesitant artists started creating. Art does not have to be intimidating. It can be fun and it can create new tools for future sensory stimulation groups or low-level one-on-one sessions. Color and pattern identification is a great indicator of levels of confusion and reality orientation.

Tribal Headdress

Size	**4 to 8**
Functioning	**high (lower with modifications)**
Time	**40-60 minutes**
Purpose	**self-understanding, self-expression, cultural experience**

The headdress has served the purpose of defining roles among people and in ceremony since the beginning of civilization. A quick look through history reveals ornate headdress and decoration among the early Peruvians, Native Americans, Aztecs, and Egyptians to name but a few. The purpose of the headdress was often to initialize the change of a man to a god, to represent a powerful god or person, or to honor a god. The more ornate the head piece, the more powerful the deity, or the person's place in society.

In the following process, participants are invited to create a headpiece that celebrates the glory of themselves, not a god or spirit. They are asked to consider all the best things about themselves and to celebrate that by creating an elaborate headpiece in the historic tradition of people all over the world.

Materials

the headdress template as depicted below, one per person, cut from heavyweight poster board

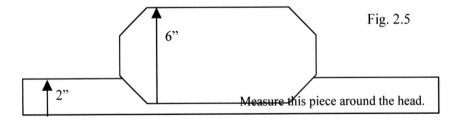

Fig. 2.5

colored or printed foam (Sax Arts and Crafts sells an
animal printed foam, call 1 800-558-6696 and ask
for item number 735-3139)
fake fur
pipe cleaners
hot glue (with supervision and hands-on assistance)
masking tape
metallic ribbons
scissors
craft (Popsicle) sticks
pictures of tribal and Peruvian headdresses (check
online, library, or *National Geographic* magazines)
mirror for viewing finished work on the participant's
head
sample headdress

Activity

1.   Start the group with photographs of traditional headdresses displayed on the table. Discuss the significance of headdresses. Ask: "Where have you seen headdresses before now?"

2.   Talk about making headdresses for themselves, in celebration of all that they have accomplished and who they are.

3.   Pass out headdress templates and measure each individual's head. Mark the spot on the headband where the band will overlap.

4.   Pass out materials and scissors. If your group members have difficulty cutting with scissors, precut the materials into more manageable pieces or assist with cutting as the process moves along.

5.   Items like pipe cleaners or ribbons may be taped with masking tape from the back of the template. All

materials could be taped or stapled to the template if necessary.

6.   Encourage the clients to have materials hang down from or expand off the top of the template. Have a sample ready to help encourage experimentation. If they have trouble getting started, help with questions such as these: "Is there an animal that you can identify with? What's your favorite color? Are you a bright person, or a dark person? Mysterious or open?"

7.   Allow 20 minutes to work; play music from other cultures if you would like to enhance the mood.

8.   When headpieces are complete, assist clients with putting on the piece, tape headband in place around the head. If the top part of the headdress is too "floppy," tape a craft stick to the back to help strengthen it.

End the group with a discussion of the various headdresses. What was each artist trying to portray about himself/herself with his/her creation? What impression would you get about the person wearing the headdress if you didn't know him/her personally? What might an archeologist of the future think of these headdresses if s/he should discover them? I guarantee you will get some interesting answers!

This group can also be done with lower cognitive functioning clients, with more hands-on assistance and some precut materials. Approach the group in a less "historic" manner and encourage the clients to experiment with the materials provided to create a "crazy hat." The tactile stimulation is great and clients generally seem to have fun with creating "hats" and seeing each other in them. Make sure you bring a mirror and encourage the artists to attempt to strike a dignified pose in their new headwear!

Stepping Stones

Size	**4 to 10**
Functioning	**high**
Time	**40-60 minutes (or more)**
Purpose	**self-understanding, long-term memory, reminiscing**

When we cross treacherous waters, when we hike through marshy grasslands, when we go from one place to another in our lives, we use stepping-stones. Every transition, change, and development in our lives requires us to take a step forward, and sometimes back. A decision is often made on faith, hope, and courage, for better or worse.

I use the stepping stone image in the following process as a lifeline tool. I ask high to medium level functioning clients to look at their lives, from youth to the present, and symbolize their journey by using stepping-stones.

Materials

construction paper in gray, blue, green, yellow, black, and red
drawing paper 24" x 14"
glue sticks
black markers
scissors

Preparation

1. Cut the gray construction paper into round-ish shapes to resemble stones.

2.   Cut the red construction paper into 14" x 4" strips to resemble flames. Like this:

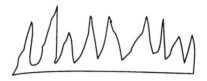

Fig 2.6

3.   Cut 14" x 4" strips of blue construction paper to resemble waves. Similar to this:

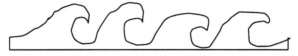

Fig 2.7

4.   Cut yellow construction paper into shapes like this:

Fig 2.8

5.   Cut green and black construction paper into 14" x 4" rectangular strips

Activity

1.   Talk about stepping-stones as described above.

2.   Distribute gray construction paper stones (start with 4 per person), and black markers.

3.   Ask each person to think of at least 4 significant points in their lives where they had to make conscious choices

about something. Suggest thinking of young adulthood (16 - 20 years of age), early adulthood (20 - 30 years of age), mid adulthood, and late adulthood. Divide up the years according to the general age group you are working with.

4. Instruct members to write one word that describes the decision that was made onto each gray stone.

5. Next, place the different colors and shapes of construction paper onto the worktable. Discuss what each color and shape can symbolize.

    •   Red = flames, which would indicate a very volatile time or a period of "hot" emotions.

    •   Green = calm pastures. Indicates smooth sailing, restful time.

    •   Black = solemn or sad times.

    •   Blue = wave shapes. Indicates rough waters, indecisive times, periods of confusion and upheaval.

    •   Yellow = sunshine and bright days. Things are good and happy.

6. Ask members to choose a color and shape for each different stone, for each different decision.

7. Next, place drawing paper in front of participants. Ask them to chronologically place the different colors of paper on the background piece as in Figure 2.9.

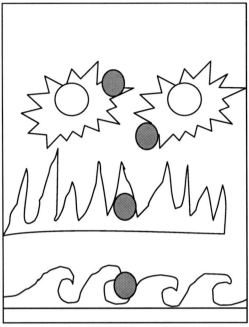

Fig 2.9

8.   Once glued in place, clients may glue the proper stepping-stone on top of the colored construction paper road.

The final piece should be a chronological map of the past years of the client's life. Discuss the visual effect of the stepping stone image. Allow each person to talk about the decisions s/he has made on the journey. Talk about how each decision affects the next. Allow ample time for processing of the stepping stone charts.

Chapter Three

Painting

Supply Selection

When looking at supplies for painting remember this: You get what you pay for. If you need to skimp with painting supplies, do it in the paper grade, not in the paints or brushes.

Paintbrushes come in a variety of widths, fibers, and some are specifically designed for specific types of paint. Avoid the student grade camel hair brushes because bristle loss and rusting is frustrating for artists and require frequent replacement, minimizing the initial cost savings. Even though your clients may not treat the brushes with the type of respect they deserve, you will alleviate a lot of frustration from your clients by not having to go through the brush-hair-pick-off adventure. Purchase some nice quality synthetic brushes in a variety of sizes and tips. These will last longer and offer your clients more success than the less expensive types of brushes.

Paint quality varies greatly in the world of watercolor paints. Avoid the bottom of the line "kiddie trays" with the ovals of concentrated paints and spend more for the higher grade paint trays, or just get really good acrylics and water them down as necessary. If you can afford them, get the nicer watercolors in a tube to be dispensed with frugality by the instructor.

Student grade watercolor paper works fine for most of the processes you do with you clients. Avoid the heavily textured papers with the bigger price tags. As good as they are for some things, for your average artist/client, they may actually take away from the intention of the application of color and make the process more difficult than necessary.

Always have paper towels and spray bottles of water handy for clean up and wetting the paper when you are away from an art area with a sink. Get some plain colored plastic table coverings to work on also. Avoid hand me down tablecloths with patterns on them. An artist may get lost in the patterns *around* their art piece rather than the patterns they are creating, and it makes materials hard to find on the tabletop.

Painting is a less desirable technique to use with lower level clients than collage for the most part, unless it is done in an abstract manner. Clients functioning at lower cognitive levels will get frustrated with the messiness and the difficulty in controlling the paint as opposed to using collage techniques where placement of paper or material is more easily achieved. Painting is also a multi-task art medium. You must 1. wet the brush, 2. dip it in paint, 3. apply it to the paper, and repeat. Many times you will find clients with some confusion skipping a step, or worse, forgetting that it is a paintbrush in their hand and not a fork or spoon. Obviously, use non-toxic materials whenever possible or when direct one-on-one supervision is not possible.

Posters

Size	**4 to 8**
Functioning	**medium (lower with adaptations)**
Time	**40-60 minutes**
Purpose	**communication, group interactions**

Look around you. Every wall, window, and bulletin board is littered with some sort of poster or flyer. Lost dogs, campaign portraits, and public health announcements are brought to us in full color, photographically, or graphically, to capture our attention on a busy day. Posters are both an advertising tool and a work of art, expressing common opinions or individual creeds. In the following process, I ask some medium cognitive/physical functioning level clients to think about posters as a communication device. Haven't they got something important to say?

Materials

> heavy-duty poster board in a variety of bright colors
>> (also referred to as railroad board by some
>> distributors) cut into 11" x 14" sheets
> acrylic paints
> large stiff brushes or sponge brushes

Activity

1. Begin discussion as stated above. Ask: "What kind of posters are you familiar with? Do you see any around the facility? What is the purpose of a poster? How do they get your attention? (bright colors, interesting images)"

2. Ask them to think of a point or thought that they would like to get across to others. It could be a philosophy, a

lesson they have learned, etc. Discuss how they might illustrate that thought.

3. Distribute supplies. Ask them to choose a colorful background for their poster.

4. Allow them 20 minutes to create their poster. First ask them to create the eye-catching background. Then, with black paint, write out the "slogan."

5. After all are complete, look at each one. Discuss how the artist got your attention with the colors or images. Discuss the thought behind the poster.

6. Display with a note on the process.

This process can also be done as a group with lower level functioning clients. Focus on the creation of a background, one color per client. Use hand over hand technique to help apply the paint. Ask questions regarding the color and shape of the image. As a group, choose a theme or idea they feel is important to them, a thought they'd like to share.

Write the theme over the background created by the group.

Script and Soul

Size	4 to 12
Functioning	medium to high
Time	30-60 minutes
Purpose	self-expression, communication

The use of the written word in art images should never be underestimated. It can take an abstract color image and make it into a concrete emotional statement. The following process pairs these two aspects to assist long-term care and rehabilitation clients to express a thought or emotion both in color and script.

Materials

list of words described in the next section
watercolor paper, 8" x 11"
spray water bottles
watercolor paints or colored inks
paintbrushes
water containers
paper towels
glue sticks

Preparation

Create a list of words that may have some significance to your client population, e.g., children, friends, love, laughter, loneliness. Write out these words or generate them on your computer, enlarging them to a size approximately 3" tall. Cut the words out of the paper. Do not cut the words into pieces.

Here are some words for you to use: Family, Friends, Health, Children, Loneliness, Hope, Laughter, Solitude, Peace, Dreams, Security, Contentment, Flight, Success, Reaching Out, Home.

Activity

1. Begin the group by discussing the development of writing. Discuss the notion that written words are merely symbols of feelings, stories, or information. Discuss using the written word as part of an artistic image.

2. Have clients choose 1 or 2 words from the cutouts you provided. Place the words on the side of their work area.

3. Ask the clients to create a colorful representation of what that word or words would "look" like to them. Ask them to use colors to express the feeling or the "soul" of the word. Encourage them to fill the whole paper surface with color in an unplanned and spontaneous way.

4. Spray paper with water to let colors flow more freely.

5. Allow 15 minutes to work.

6. Once complete, absorb some of the excess water with paper towels and have clients place their words on the image.

7. Apply glue and secure. You may need to wait until the paper dries before you glue the words onto the painting.

8. Review images. Ask: "Does the use of the written word enhance the visual image or detract from it? Do you feel the words and the colors used reflect each other accurately? Why did you choose the specific words used in your images?"

9. Matte or mount pieces onto black poster or matte board and display.

Cultural Flags

Size	**4 to 8**
Functioning	**medium to high**
Time	**40-60 minutes**
Purpose	**reminiscing, self-worth, long-term memory**

Individuals are made up of so many infinite factors; our family, friends, and cultural backgrounds all combine to affect our personal characteristics and beliefs. Most people associate to some extent with their original ethnic heritage, so many possibilities, each country with its own language, culture, and flags.

The following process was developed to help foster a sense of the historical self, a sense of the individual, as well as an opportunity to discuss ethnic backgrounds and share them with each other.

Materials

> a reference source that includes color representations of the many different country flags (an encyclopedia generally has this, or go to your local library and check reference books on flags and atlases)
> acrylic paints
> brushes
> white painting paper approximately 8" x 14"
> paint trays
> water buckets
> paper towels

Activity

1.
> Discuss ethnic and cultural backgrounds of the participants. As they identify their heritage, show them

pictures of their respective country's flags. Perhaps tell them a little bit about the country, e.g., historical events and other interesting information, or have them tell you what they know!

2. Distribute art materials. Discuss the impact of our heritage on our upbringing, how they developed as individuals.

3. Using *only* the colors of the flag of their country, ask them to create a flag of their own that may represent something about their background both ethnically and personally. Have them create a flag that would reflect individual characteristics as well as important cultural images. The flag can be abstract or representational.

4. Allow 20 minutes to work.

5. When all are complete, discuss the images. Ask: "Did the limitation of using the flag's colors hamper your abilities to create an accurate interpretation of your own flag? How does your flag represent you? What kind of feeling did the original flag instill upon you and how did that change?"

End the group with a discussion of the language of their countries. If possible, exchange good-byes in their different languages.

Sometimes it is refreshing to touch base with our own history and the history of our families. This process may open up discussion of many family memories: immigration, strife, and success that make up the pride we feel in being who we are.

Mono Prints

Size	4 to 8
Functioning	**any**
Time	**20-60 minutes**
Purpose	**gross motor movement, self-expression, relaxation, abstract thinking**

There is something innately soothing about images in motion. Waves upon the water, birds flying gracefully in the blue sky, tropical fish in a softly lit tank, all these things elicit an almost hypnotic response. This allows us to block out the clutter of the day, let go of our concerns, and just enjoy the experience.

Color in motion creates the same response. The use of flowing paints, moving together over a smooth surface, allows us to let go of our need to create an image, and to just create.

The method used in this process is a combination of finger painting and mono printing, combined to offer the opportunity for the clients to lose themselves in an aesthetic and tactile creative event.

Materials

plastic table covering (of shower curtain weight)

finger paint paper, 11" x 16" (or use freezer wrap, shiny side up, although paper will eventually curl)

finger paints or watered-down acrylics (hand lotion consistency)

plastic gloves

palette knives

brayers (hand-inking rollers)

water source for clean up

melodic music of your choice

Preparation

1.   Cover surface of table with plastic covering. This will be your painting surface.

Activity

1.   Begin group with a discussion of the soothing qualities of objects in motion as described in the introduction. Can they think of any other examples?

2.   Invite them to experience art making as a soothing process. Ask them to listen to the music, or to the rhythm of themselves, and apply paints to the plastic sheeting using hands, fingers, knives, or whatever. Encourage them to stretch their arms, to "dance" with the paint across the table. No planned images, just move and blend the colors. Start music.

3.   As work slows, look at areas of their images to print from.

4.   Apply slick paper over the surface of the table and rub it down with hand or brayer.

5.   Remove prints and allow them to dry.

6.   When all are through, discuss how music affected their movement. Ask: "Were you able to enjoy the movement of the paint, without worrying about the images or the textures? Were you able to clear your heads? Did you feel a sense of relaxation?"

7.   Review the prints. Title each print and matte or mount as you wish.

Your musical choice will make a big difference in the tone of the artwork. I use new age type music, something mellow and light.

"All the World's a Stage"

Size	**4 to 8**
Functioning	**medium to high (low with modifications)**
Time	**40-60 minutes**
Purpose	**life review, reminiscing**

We are a society of cinema lovers. We love our movies. The type of movies we are drawn to say something about our personality. This process asks you to open a discussion about movies with your clients. Find out what their favorite movies are, and why. Begin to move the discussion to their own lives. What kind of movie would their life be, and how can they reflect that movie through artistic means.

Materials

11" x 17" white drawing paper

craypas or markers

pictures of movie posters that your client population would be familiar with, e.g., *Gone with the Wind* for seniors, Disney movies for children

Activity

1. Begin with a discussion of favorite movies. Ask each person to name his/her favorite movie, and say why s/he liked it. As you go around the group, determine what genre the movie fits into. Ask: "What about that type of movie appeals to you?"

2. Next ask group members to think about a most memorable moment of their own lives. Which of their

	personal experiences do they think would make a great movie?
3.	Go around the group and offer the opportunity to discuss their chosen memory.
4.	Next ask them to create a movie title to summarize the event.
5.	Finally, ask them to create a movie poster to "advertise" the film.
6.	Pass out markers, craypas, and paper. Instruct participants to use these items to create their own posters. Ask them to think about the images that come to mind when they think of the event, and to pick one or several of these images to recreate.

There are other ways to go with the movie theme, depending on the cognitive and cohesive level of the group. Instead of totally creating a film from their own experiences, you can ask the group members to chose a film title that they feel reflects something about their lives. Have several titles in mind ahead of time to help narrow down the choices, e.g., *Gone with the Wind*, *On Golden Pond*, *Casablanca*, and *True Grit* for seniors or *Nightmare on Elm Street*, *Cinderella*, *Star Wars*, and *Mission Impossible* for younger participants. Then, offer the opportunity to discuss how the title reflects their lives and create a movie poster reflecting that "scene." If your clients are hesitant to create a poster from scratch, offer cut pictures from magazines, look for large pictures and images of people.

One last way to touch on the movie theme with lower level clients is to offer collage pictures and words. Have them create a theme-based collage; then create a "title" for the scene that is portrayed.

A great portion of this process is the discussion that goes along with it. Don't rush or underestimate the importance of the discussion and the potential to do some life review.

Body Painting and Tattoos

Size	**4 to 10**
Functioning	**high**
Time	**40-60 minutes**
Purpose	**self-expression, trust building**

Tattoos have become very popular within the last few years. Most young adults have a tattoo (or piercing) somewhere on their body. Generally tattoos are done in an effort to express something about oneself.

Historically, tattoos have been part of various rites of passage. Some cultures begin the tattoo process on boys as a symbolic representation of that boy's transition into manhood. Many a Marine or other US Armed Service person has used a tattoo of an eagle or a flag to express his love for his country. There have even been a few men and women out there that have had their loved one's name tattooed on their body as a symbol of everlasting love.

The following process looks at the tattoo in a fun way, discussing its history, and giving high cognitive functioning level clients the opportunity to express themselves in a non-permanent way. This process also calls for individuals to pair off and paint on each other. This challenges their trust in fellow group members, and enhances the feeling that the group works together towards common goals.

Materials

> face or body paints (available through your area craft shop, or costume and party store)
> small water buckets
> paper towels
> scrap paper
> small paintbrushes
> samples of tattoos that would be appropriate

Activity

1.   To begin, talk about tattoos. Ask: "Does anyone in the group have one? What are your feelings about tattoos?" Discuss body painting in different cultures (war paint, tribal art patterns). Talk about how body art has been used as a rite of passage. Discuss some of the examples given above. If possible, encourage clients or staff that have tattoos to share their tattoos with the group and to discuss their reasons for getting the tattoo.

2.   Look at samples of tattoo-type symbols and drawings. Find pictures that are common to tattoos (for example, roses, skull and cross bones, eagle). Discuss the different types of meanings these could hold.

3.   Ask each person to think about something that is important to him/her. How could s/he symbolize that in the form of a body tattoo?

4.   Pass out body paints. Pass out brushes, water, paper towels, and scrap paper to practice on.

5.   Pair off individuals. If you have an odd number, feel free to join in. Instruct them to share ideas with each other about what kind of tattoo they would like. Have them work as a team to do the other's tattoo. Encourage them to choose simple shapes or symbols, and to practice on the paper before painting each other.

6.   Tattoos will be painted on the forearm of the client, unless otherwise (and appropriately) requested. Other places can be the top of the hand, the upper arm, or face. Most body paints are non-toxic so the face and hands would be all right.

7.   Using the small paintbrushes, clients may begin taking turns painting on the other's tattoo.

8.   When done, allow the tattoos to dry as clients are encouraged to share the story of their tattoo.

9.   To close the session, talk about permanent tattoos. Would any of them have been brave enough to have it permanently done?

Overall, this session is fun oriented, with the discussion portion being just as important as the art process. It is meant to encourage clients to think about what is really of the most importance to them. Many clients will paint a loved one's name on their arm, or their spouse's favorite flower to express love.

NOTE: I have not forgotten that tattoos have negative connotations also, for example the tattooing of Holocaust victims arms with numbers. If possible, steer away from this use of tattoos. Be sensitive to your client's history. If you have clients in your group who have personal experiences with the Holocaust and you feel they will react to this process in a negative way, use this process as a "body painting" group and skip the tattoo background and history.

Independence Day

Size	**4 to 8**
Functioning	**high**
Time	**two 40-60 minute sessions**
Purpose	**independence, self-expression, self-worth**

We celebrate our independence, especially in July. It is a time when we think about sacrifices and freedom in many different ways. Overall, if asked on July 4th, your basic American would reply to the question, "Are you free?" with a "Yes." However, freedom is not a word many seniors or individuals living in a controlled environment would agree describes their lifestyle.

When entering a nursing home or rehab center, the "patients" give themselves over to someone else's rules, giving up their freedom in a lot of ways.

The following process leads group members in a discussion of freedom, focusing on issues of personal freedom, or the quest for greater control and independence. This is a two-group process.

Materials

sheets of student grade watercolor paper, 2 sheets per person, approximately 8" x 11"
water spray bottles
table coverings or work trays
glue sticks
paper towels
pencils
scissors
colored ink in bottles with eyedroppers (such as Dr. Martin Bombay India Ink available through Sax Arts

and Crafts or Design Higgins® India Ink from Nasco.)

Activity

1.   Begin the group with a discussion of independence. Ask them to define the word. Ask: "How are you independent?" Discuss the ways we can be independent even under circumstances that force us to be somewhat dependent.

2.   Discuss the word "freedom." Ask: "How are you free? What do you perceive are things that take away your freedom? How can you maintain your freedoms — the ways you are free?"

3.   Place one sheet of watercolor paper in front of each person. Saturate it with water, either by spray bottle or by dipping it in a tray of water.

4.   Ask members to think about their personal definition of independence. Ask them to think about the ways they are independent and to choose colors that might reflect their feelings of independence.

5.   Drop colored ink onto the wet paper. Spray paper with more water to blend colors. Ask the artists to fill the entire paper with colors.

6.   Move these papers aside; absorb ink puddles on the paper with paper towels. Wipe the table area clean of spilled ink.

7.   Place a clean, wet sheet of paper in front of each person.

8.   Ask them to consider their personal definition of freedom. Ask them to think of how they are free. (If your group members feel strongly that they are in *no* way free, that is okay. Ask them to choose colors that

reflect that feeling of non-freedom, if that's how they feel the strongest.)

9.   Use the inks in the same way as step #5.

10.   Allow sheets to dry until the next group time.

At the next meeting time, place both dried sheets of inked paper in front of the artist who created them.

1.   Ask them to choose one sheet to keep whole, as a background, and one sheet that will be cut or torn.

2.   Tell group members that they are to create a "flag" with the papers they made in the last group.

3.   Ask members to think about what symbols or shapes they may like to create that may reflect something about how they feel independence and freedom relate to them. How they "feel" their independence and freedom.

4.   Using the scissors, or by tearing, allow the participants to create forms, either representative or symbolic to attach to their "flag." Some may choose stripes or stars like the American flag, and that is fine as long as they can explain what that says to them, how it expresses something about their individuality, or how they relate to America.

5.   Glue forms in place.

Discuss overall impressions of the flags. Do the artists feel they accurately represent the way they feel, positive or negatively about their independence and freedom? For those members who are completely frustrated and feel they have no control over their environment, remind them of how they can experience independence.

It is important to remind the participants in your art group that independence and freedom are extremely personal things. That only they can control their thoughts and feelings. Only they themselves can choose to be active or inactive, to choose to continue to learn, to grow, to continue to experience new things in spite of their challenges. And remind them especially that as long as they choose, they have the freedom to express themselves through art.

Chapter Four

Drawing

Materials and Age Appropriateness

As discussed in Chapter One of this book, the materials one selects to work with are just as important as the processes they are used in. Drawing materials can vary from expensive colored pencils, to crayons. The way the materials are perceived, as well as how they perform, are very important when presenting them to your clients.

I try to use oil pastels instead of wax crayons whenever possible only because crayons are perceived as "kid's toys" by teens and adults and quickly raise a red flag in the hesitant artist's mind.

Creating art does not come naturally to many people. Therefore it is imperative that you introduce them to the materials in a respectful and professional manner.

Avoid smudgy chalks or charcoal pencils for drawings, as the unintended smudges will frustrate your clients and give them an excuse to give up. Opt for smudge free pencils or markers when asking them to draw. Remember, materials are half the success of a project. Presentation is the other, which I will discuss at the end of this book.

Drawing methods are best when you really want the clients to think about the challenge of the process. Drawing also allows them the most opportunity for self-evaluation and discovery. It is also, by far, the easiest material to take into a day room or for a one-on-one meeting. Higher-level cognitive functioning clients find it a little more time consuming, but it offers more control over line or color placement. While they work for small projects, drawing tools such as oil pastels or drawing pencils are nor suitable for large, abstract art. Drawing tools take far too long in the kind of projects where you want instant color and movement. Refer to the chart at the beginning of this book for more information on the nature of drawing.

Rejuvenation

Size	**4 to 10**
Functioning	**high**
Time	**40-60 minutes**
Purpose	**renewal, hopefulness, reminiscing**

Springtime is a time where evidence of the earth's ability to be reborn and rejuvenated is all around us. Every year, despite the ravages of winter, the scars from the past seasons seem to be forgotten as we greet the newness of our surroundings. This process need not be limited to nature's beauty but, with some creativity, can be applied to us also. Before we can be ready to be "reborn," we need to address the issues of our past. Here's how:

Materials

        drawing paper (8" x 11")
        markers
        oil pastels or crayons
        black construction paper (8" x 11")
        glue sticks
        scissors (optional)

Activity

1.   Discuss rebirth. Ask: "What does it mean to you? How do you see the miracle of rebirth or rejuvenation in the world?"

2.   Ask the participants to think of their own ability to be rejuvenated. Ask: "Is it possible for us to refresh ourselves, to, in essence, be reborn?"

3.   Instruct the group to create an image of their past on the drawing paper. Using colors, images, or words they can depict significant events both good and bad. Allow 10 minutes to work.

4.   Remove markers and crayons and place the black construction paper and glue sticks on the table.

5.   Talk about rebirth. In order to refresh ourselves, to feel renewed, we must move away from our past, taking the good and the bad and learning from it, to create a new future.

6.   Ask the group members to create a new image from the old. Have them tear their first image into pieces of various shapes (or cut with scissors if they prefer).

        For clients that have difficulty with this, remind them that they are not losing the beauty of their first image, but merely changing it into something new. This is also the reason I only allow 10 minutes to create this image. Limiting the time spent creating the image can also limit their attachment to the artwork.

7.   Using the glue sticks, create a collage on the black paper with the torn pieces.

8.   When finished, look at the final products. Ask your clients to reflect upon them. Can they give them titles?

Finish the group with a discussion of how the events and feelings of our past affect and shape our future. We always need to creatively look at our good times and bad times, and find beauty in it all.

Creativity vs. Logic

Size	**4 to 10**
Functioning	**high (medium with modifications)**
Time	**40-60 minutes**
Purpose	**abstract thinking, self-discovery, communication**

A self-portrait can be defined in many ways. It can be a realistic representation of the person, or it can be a collage of memories, feelings, and experiences. However you choose to portray yourself, the act of self-portrayal is done to gain a better understanding of who we are to ourselves, as well as to others.

The following process looks at two very specific aspects of the self in a self-portrait format. Here we focus on the hemispherical division of the brain. Are we more of a creative thinker or a logical thinker?

Materials

drawing paper
craypas or markers
black markers
paper weights
pre drawn portrait heads (Fig. 4.1)
glue sticks

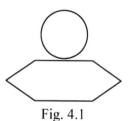

Fig. 4.1

Preparation

1.   Draw the paper heads on 11" x 15" drawing paper.

Activity

1.   Discuss the difference between logical thinking and creative thinking. Ask: "What type of thinking do you do

best? Are you more logical and scientific, or are you more creative and spontaneous?"

2.   Distribute the paper with the portrait head silhouettes to each person.

3.   Ask your clients to divide their portrait into the two parts discussed, the creative and the logical. Ask them to make a line, curvy or straight, to divide the silhouette into two parts. They should leave more room for the part that they feel is more significant for them.

4.   Encourage them to then create images of what these two parts, the logical and the creative, would look like to them. Ask: "How are you creative? How are you logical or scientific?"

5.   Allow 20 minutes to work.

6.   When finished, review the work. Discuss their decisions about what kind of thinker they are. Ask: "Does it matter if you are a man or a woman? Can you be equally creative and logical? Do you wish you were more of one than the other?"

An adaptation of this process can be used with lower level clients using magazine pictures and words cut out ahead of time by you. Provide the portrait silhouette to your clients; ask them to create an image of themselves using the collage materials. Provide photos that may stir memories or point to meaningful issues in their lives, such as homes, children, families, tools, boots (to represent work for the men), etc. Make sure pictures and words are large enough to be seen by clients with poor vision. Assist them in selecting images that have meaning to them and encourage story sharing as the group progresses. Glue onto paper using glue sticks.

Renewal

Size	4 to 8
Functioning	high
Time	40-60 minutes
Purpose	remotivation, self-discovery, communication, life review

Trees are often used as markers of time. They tell a story to the viewer about their environment, the history of their lives, and what the world has been like around them. Their resiliency in spite of their experiences is inspirational.

The tree image is traditionally a significant image of the self in art therapy. We can relate to its organic qualities, as well as to its abilities to change and be affected by changing circumstances. We, like the trees, can continue to grow.

Materials

drawing paper (11" x 15")
crayons or craypas or wide tip markers

Preparation

1. Separate the crayons or markers with brown and black in one group and the rest of the colors in a second group.

Activity

1. Begin the group with a discussion of trees, their nature, and symbolic meanings to us. Ask the group to imagine themselves as trees.

2. Pass out the brown and black markers. Talk about how trees renew themselves with the seasons' changing

environment, how the dormant season always gives way to spring and new growth. Ask group members to draw their tree as it appears in winter.

3.   When done, place the other colors on the tables. Ask the participants to look ahead to seasons of renewal. Think about the possibilities ahead, how the changes of the season and the passage of time may affect them and what opportunities may be presented to them.

4.   Have them imagine those possibilities as colors, as movement of lines. Ask them to create the crown of the tree and the areas around the tree using the colors and lines that would best represent how they see changes ahead and the emotions and feeling they may experience.

5.   Allow 20 minutes to work.

6.   When all are complete, look at the individual pictures. Ask: "What kind of feeling does the viewer get from looking at it? Can we guess about what the artist may predict for the future?"

7.   Then ask the clients to describe what is represented in their pictures. Are they imagining positive things, negative things, or both occurring in the future?

Spontaneously, other group members may offer words of comfort and optimism to those with more negative outlooks. You may want to discuss the philosophy that life always seems to provide us with a mixture of good and bad times. The hard times help us to appreciate the good.

When doing a group like this always be prepared to deal with the issues of your clients. Think ahead about the issues you know the individuals in your group are going through and whether or not it would be helpful and appropriate to implement a group of this kind.

It may also be useful to have a sample to show ahead of time to help break the clients away from the strictly conventional and realistic representation of trees and landscapes with traditional colors. It sometimes helps to free them from the nagging thoughts of "Am I doing this right?"

Create one for yourself. How does your tree grow?

The Cards You Are Dealt

Size	**4 to 10**
Functioning	**high (options for lower)**
Time	**40-60 minutes**
Purpose	**life review, self-discovery, remotivation**

We have all heard the expression, "You have to play the game of life with the cards you have been dealt." What if we could change the character and emotion of the playing deck? What if "disasters or hardships" were seen as "challenges?" What if "regrets" were viewed as "wisdom?" What kind of hand could we play with if the nature of our cards were different?

Using new materials available, we can have some fun with the creation of our own special playing cards!

Materials

blank set of playing cards available through Sax Arts and Crafts catalog (1-800-558-6696)
permanent markers in a variety of colors and point widths.

Activity

1. Begin the group by asking participants how the game of cards relates to life. Phrases like "You have to play the cards you have been dealt." Or "You've got to know when to hold 'em, know when to fold 'em" are two of the commonly known references you may hear. Ask: "What does that mean to you?"

2.　　　　Divide the cards equally among group members. Each member should have at least 5 cards to enhance.

3.　　　　One side of the cards is decorated. Ask the participants to think about some of the cards they have been dealt, good and bad, and encourage them to create images of these events or situations on the blank side of the card. If you want to keep the mood of the group lighter, ask them to create a "hand" of their own choice. For example, they may decide that they would like to win the lottery and travel; they would then create "wish cards."

4.　　　　Encourage use of the entire blank area. The phrase "cover all the white" sometimes helps participants think more about their image making.

5.　　　　Make sure card makers initial their artwork. They can write one word on the top of the card to describe the kind of emotion the card details. For example, one person may have been dealt a card related to the birth of a child. The card is done in pink, as it is a girl, along with other images of the participant's daughter. The artist might write the word "Joy" on the top of the card.

6.　　　　When their allotted cards have been decorated, ask the participants to hold them in their hands as if they were going to play poker. Ask: "What is the overall tone of the hand? Do you feel you could 'win' with the hand you have been dealt?" If the artist represented the cards s/he felt s/he *has* been dealt, did the artist focus only on negative situations? Or was s/he able to see the bright side of the cards also? (Remind them that the ace can be both the lowest card in the deck and the highest. It all depends what game you are playing or how you use it.)

7.　　　　At the end of the session, allow the artists to either take their cards home or to keep them together as a group deck. If you keep the cards together, use them with other groups for some of the processes discussed below.

Options

1.   Lower level groups can identify colors or emotions expressed on cards that are picked from the deck.

2.   Higher-level groups can pick a card at random and use it as inspiration for a drawing or painting. Ask them to look at the card and imagine a story to go behind it or to determine the meaning of the card to them.

3.   Place like card themes together, visually showing how we all share similar experiences.

All in all, participants should leave the group reminded that the cards of life are shuffled often and, if we feel our luck has been poor, the next shuffle may bring us greater fortune.

"Top Secret"

Size	**4 to 8**
Functioning	**high**
Time	**40-60 minutes**
Purpose	**life review, trust, group interaction**

Anyone who has ever seen any kind of spy movie knows that someone snooping around will eventually make his/her way to a file cabinet and pull out the conspicuously marked "TOP SECRET" folder.

According to movies, and your high school principal, all the interesting and compelling information about each one of us is held in such a folder in *somebody's* file cabinet.

The following process takes a lighthearted look at what each of us imagines someone may find upon discovering our secret folder. The program leader may ask the group to look at the process seriously or in a "Just for Fun" manner, depending on the group, their dynamics, and their willingness to open up to others.

Warning: Do not use this process when dealing with clients who tend towards paranoia or who are significantly confused.

Materials

          office type, manila file folders — the kind that open and lay flat — one per person
          oil pastels or markers
          black markers

Optional

          collage materials like lace fabric
          words and pictures cut from magazines
          scissors
          glue sticks (solid not liquid)

Preparation

1.   Prepare each folder by writing "TOP SECRET" across
                the front.

2.   Cut words and pictures from magazines that can be
                placed in the folder.

Activity

1.   Place one folder in front of each person.

2.   Introduce the group much as I have above. Ask: "If you
                were to create your own TOP SECRET file, what kind
                of information would you put into it?"

                •   For the lighthearted group: ask members to
                        create images inside the folder to represent some
                        of their most interesting adventures, their secret
                        nicknames, or most embarrassing moments. Let
                        them know they do not have to share the
                        information in the folder and that they should
                        only create images or symbols of these things.
                        Optional: use collage materials to symbolize the
                        contents of their file.

                •   For the more serious group: ask members to
                        think of the things they hold in their hearts: the
                        memories, the thoughts, and ideas that they have
                        had that they share only with close friends, or
                        maybe with no one at all. Ask them to use color
                        or symbols to create images inside the folder to
                        represent these things. Again, let them know that
                        these are for their eyes only and that they do not
                        need to share their images with anyone if they
                        do not want to. This should only be done with
                        high-level clients whom you know well. You
                        don't want to scare group members away if they

have not bonded with you or other group members.

3.   If group members have a hard time starting, help them out with some examples. For instance, for the lighthearted group, tell them something you may have in your file, like a grade school nickname. For the more serious group, share a fear, or a secret, like you stuttered as a kid or you pushed your sister off the swing set (Sorry Sis!).

4.   When all have completed their files, offer everyone the chance to talk about some or all of the contents.

5.   Then as the group ends, offer the group the option of keeping their files with them or tearing them up and throwing them away so no one else can look into their file. Thank them for investigating their files with you.

This process offers individuals a chance to do some life review in a fun way or in a more serious manner, using non-threatening materials. The file folder offers immediate privacy, by allowing the artist to close his file or reveal its contents as s/he chooses. I recommend doing a file for yourself with the group, to allow them to see you sharing your ideas with them as they do with you. By participating along with them, you reinforce the safety of the process and the feeling of group cohesiveness.

Guardians

Size	**4 to 8**
Functioning	**high (medium with modifications)**
Time	**40-60 minutes**
Purpose	**self-discovery, group dynamics, self-worth**

The myth of the spiritual guardian has been around for centuries. Popular Roman myth called them Genius and Juno, creative spirits who would watch over us from birth to death. Native Americans have attributed their inner guidance to animal spirits that watch over and protect them. Popular now is the belief in guardian angels, which, many believe, help us through crises in our lives.

In any culture, at any point in history, these mysterious guardians are credited with preserving our safety, bringing us luck and happiness.

The following process asks the participants to think about their beliefs in reference to guardians and to create an image of what that being might look like to them.

Materials

drawing paper
markers

Preparation

1. For use with lower level clients, draw a figure template on the paper to help get them started.

Activity

1. Discuss the mythology of guardian spirits. Ask: "What do you believe? Do you feel you have a guardian?"

2.   Whatever their beliefs, ask them to create, in their minds, an image of what their guardian would look like. Ask them to consider the following attributes when "designing" him/her.

- Does your guardian need to be strong, quick, wise, peaceful? What attributes do you feel a guardian spirit could have that would benefit you.

- Is it male or female? Why?

- Does it lead you or follow behind as support?

- Does it have any special powers?

3.   Ask them to write down any attributes they think their guardian would have on the top of the paper.

4.   Invite them to begin to draw the image they have in mind on the drawing paper. Lower level clients would draw over or "dress" the template form provided.

5.   As participants begin to finish the main image, ask them if their guardian has any special tools, weapons, or powers that they could draw.

6.   When all are complete, discuss the images. Ask: "What attributes does your guardian have? Why did you select them? What are some of the things your guardian would have to do for you?" If their guardian has any tools or implements, refer to those for explanation.

The processing part of this group may bring a lot of laughter, or may be taken more seriously, depending on the mood of your group. In either case, the creation of a guardian can bring insight into what a person feels are his/her weaknesses or what type of insecurities an individual may have.

Close the group with a discussion of what our perceived fears are and why people are thankful to have guardians. Remind group members that their circle of friends and family members are often composed of a number of our best "guardians," people who look out for us. Each person that touches our lives in a positive way is a guardian to our self-esteem and self-worth.

We are all guardians to each other.

The Golden Rule

Size	**4 to 8**
Functioning	**high (low with modifications)**
Time	**40-60 minutes**
Purpose	**life review, socialization**

We have all heard of the Golden Rule: "Do unto others as you would have them do unto you," or "Harm no one." The Golden Rule is loosely applied to a philosophy of life. The following process asks artists to think about their own philosophy of life, their own Golden Rule, and to express it both in words and in color and shape.

Using a new product offered by Sax Arts and Crafts makes this process fun and unusual, even though the topic may have been broached before.

Materials

clear 12" rulers with snap in panel available through
    Nasco (800) 558-9595
permanent markers in a variety of colors
scrap pieces of paper
cellophane tape

Activity

1.   Discuss the term, "The Golden Rule." Ask: "What is your personal Golden Rule or philosophy of life?"

2.   Distribute materials and ask members to decorate their ruler insert with images or colors that express the feeling behind their philosophy. Ask them not to write words at this point.

Tape the insert down onto blank scrap paper of a darker color so that individuals can work to the edge of the insert without worrying about drawing on the table. The bigger backdrop piece also offers more surface to hold onto when drawing. Make sure they understand that the scrap paper is just a tool and will not be part of their finished image.

3.   When images are done, ask participants if they would like to write their philosophy over their image. (You can help with this, to make sure the words are easy to read). Have each artist sign his/her work.

4.   Snap inserts into clear rulers.

5.   Allow the creators to use this ruler as a reminder of their personal Golden Rule, or to offer it to children or grandchildren so that their philosophies are passed on to future generations.

Another way to use this ruler art is to discuss feelings about "rules." Have the group discuss good rules vs. bad rules and create an image of what their feelings about rules are. Ask them to write on the insert some of the rules they are thinking about.

Chapter Five

Miscellaneous

This chapter is filled with fun, interesting plans that use unusual or hard to categorize materials. It ties the theme of the group directly to the materials that will be used. Most of the materials used can be found at local craft supply stores but, if you have trouble finding them, think creatively for substitutes, or for supplies that may fit your budget more appropriately.

Some of these processes could be considered collage, however, because of the materials or the theme, I have decided to place them here.

Many of these techniques are great team building projects. Plans like "Similarly Dissimilar," "Life Orb," and "Flying Free" are fun, active, and inspire discussion of ideas that are important for people who work together to explore. These particular processes don't require much art skill, but provide an opportunity for creativity, openness, and bonding.

Instruments of Communication

Size	**4 to 8**
Functioning	**high to medium**
Time	**40-60 minutes**
Purpose	**group dynamics, communication, self-discovery**

Heimdall, according to Norse mythology, was the "White God." A watchman, he had perfect vision, acute hearing, and could go without sleep for days. He, however, could not speak. Because of this, he was given a special horn, made for him by Odin, the God of War. This was Heimdall's only way to communicate.

This legend had me wondering how we might communicate with each other if our speech was altered or taken away. People who have speech deficits due to an accident, disease, hearing loss, or stroke sometimes deal with a great amount of frustration trying to get their needs met or understood. The following process is a challenge to clients with high to medium level functioning to communicate their needs with sounds other than that of their voice. It might be good to have an intern or volunteer to assist with this group. Clients may have trouble closing off the ends of their shakers or may need assistance in holding and manipulating their instruments as they decorate them.

Materials

        heavy weight construction paper in various colors
        acrylic paints
        small cardboard boxes (from jewelry box size to
            envelope box size, whatever can fit comfortably in
            one hand)
        wooden spoons like the type you find in a craft store

2 lbs. of dried beans
1 lb. of rice
toilet paper and paper towel rolls
colored permanent markers
clear tape
heavy rubber bands
colored masking tape

Activity

1.   Begin the group by telling the story of Heimdall. Talk about what it would be like to communicate with each other without using words. Ask: "How could you express yourself, your different emotions by using sounds instead of words?"

2.   Ask the group to think about making sound devices. Each person will create a sound maker that will help him/her to express feelings without using words. Talk about the different possibilities.

- Shakers: any kind of box or tube filled with dried beans or rice that will make noise when shaken.

- Drums: anything that will make a noise when you strike it. (Make sure they know that although striking their neighbor would most likely result in a noise, that does not mean s/he is a drum!)

3.   Place boxes and rolls on the table and talk about how to make them into instruments. Boxes will be hit with wooden spoons or with the hand; rolls will be filled with beans or rice and can be shaken.

4.   Once a box or roll has been selected, ask the clients to decorate the tubes or boxes in a way that would represent them or what they want to communicate. For

example, if the client is a very showy, vibrant person or wants to communicate in an excited way, s/he may decorate his/her instrument with bright colors and swirls.

5.   Those who selected a box to make into a drum can also choose a wooden spoon to paint or decorate as part of their instrument.

6.   Allow 10 - 15 minutes to paint or apply decoration to instruments. Assist as necessary.

7.   When outside decorations have been completed on the boxes or rolls, complete the "noise making" portion of the instrument.

- For those who selected rolls, choose a color of construction paper, and wrap one end of the roll to seal it shut. To do this, cut a circle of paper about an inch and a half larger than the opening. Put glue on the end of the tube and wrap the circle of paper over the opening so it is glued to the tube. Secure it with tape or a rubber band. Using fabric to do this also works well, although it limits the rattling sound of the noisemaker. Add beans or rice, depending on the noise the person wants to produce and seal the other end in the same manner.

- Drums may also be filled with beans or rice to add a rattling sound when hit. Seal boxes with tape or hold shut with rubber bands if filled with noisemakers.

8.   When all are complete (and you can tell this when all the noise starts!), ask them to go around the table and introduce themselves by making their own special noise.

9.   When everyone has introduced himself or herself, ask them all to make a joyful noise all at once, then an angry

noise, and then a sad noise. Talk about how those sounds changed.

End the group by saying goodbye with the instruments. Allow members to take their instruments with them, or save them as a group for future sound communications!

Your group members will really enjoy the ability to combine music and art as an alternative to communicating verbally. They also seem to enjoy the ability to just make noise. Something about being noisy makes you feel free. Try it yourself!

Planting Inspiration

Size	**4 to 8**
Functioning	**high to medium**
Time	**40-60 minutes**
Purpose	**hopefulness, rebirth, self-discovery, sensory stimulation**

Springtime is a time of nurturing and growth. We look around us to find nature beginning to show signs of rebirth and renewal. Now, it seems, is a good time to take a lesson from nature and revitalize and nourish ourselves. This is necessary in order for us to continue to be the best we can be. The following process utilizes nature elements to help connect participants with the process in nature of rebirth, nourishing, and growth.

Materials

plastic flowerpot planters with a transparent sleeve that holds a paper insert you can decorate (available through Sax Arts and Crafts 1-800-558-6696), one per participant

magic markers with the wide tip for easy coverage

potting soil

sunflower or marigold seeds

plastic gloves

plastic cups

Activity

1.   Set up the room with the markers and paper inserts on the table. Keep pots, soil, and seeds out of the way.

2. Talk about the season of spring. "April showers bring May flowers." Ask: "What do you equate with April? What kinds of things begin to happen in nature?"

3. Now generalize the conversation to growing things. Ask: "What does it take to make something grow? (water, sunshine, warmth)"

4. Begin a discussion of nurturing. "If you were going to grow something, you would have to nurture it, like a flower seed. You would have to take care of it and watch over it, give it attention so it would grow strong."

5. Next ask: "What can you nurture inside of *you* that would make you a better person? What traits or feelings would you like to develop?" As with growing a flower, to change or improve ourselves, we have to work at it, nurture ourselves. Ask them to finish this sentence: "In order to be a better person, I want to work on my ability to _____."

6. Using the paper inserts and the markers provided, invite the group to each create an image of what they want to "nurture inside of themselves." Their images can be abstract colors and movement of lines or something more representative. Ask them not to use words at this point.

7. When the inserts are finished, discuss the images. Allow each person to sum up his/her goal in one word and write that word somewhere on the insert if s/he would like to.

8. Place the inserts in plastic sleeves and put aside.

9. Next, place some newspaper on the table along with the soil, pots, and seeds. Using a plastic cup, scoop out some soil to fill the pots.

10.   Ask clients to chose some seeds and plant them in their pots.

11.   Next, slip the plastic sleeves onto the pots.

12.   End the group with a discussion on nurturing ourselves as Mother Nature nurtures her offspring at this time of the year. Talk about the importance of giving ourselves the things we need to grow as people, and to nurture our hopes, dreams, and goals, as well as the goals of our friends.

This process combines the sensory stimulation of working with soil and things of nature, self-examination, and discussion of how we can continue to grow as individuals. Small plants can be purchased to fill the pots if you fear the clients will be unable to maintain the pot to sprout a plant. Pots can also be kept in a central area for one member of the group to watch over if you have doubts about the safety and success of your seedlings. Most importantly, the artists should not feel disappointed if their seedlings do not come up. You can always incorporate the common struggles towards achieving our goals as part of your group process, in preparation for the possibility that the plants may fail to flourish.

Apple for the Teacher

Size	**4 to 8**
Functioning	**high (lower with modifications)**
Time	**40-60 minutes**
Purpose	**reminiscing, remotivation**

Reminiscence of school days is always very successful with older participants. Good or bad, they all seem to remember something about being in school and learning and playing with others. For clients who are still in school, thinking about school may bring up issues that are very hard to deal with, especially if they have suffered a significant loss of function that will impact their future schooling.

This exercise does not focus on current school situations. Instead, it looks back at the "old days" when there were no metal detectors or the necessity of deeming a school a "drug free zone." It may be real or mythical, but we believe that there was a time when students learned important lessons and respected their teachers.

The following process looks back on how school used to be and the tradition of bringing an "apple for the teacher." Wasn't that event a symbol of a student's affection for his/her teacher and a thank you for lessons learned?

Materials

        medium to large size papier-mâché or wooden apples
            available at craft supply stores, one per client
        acrylic paints
        black 3-D fabric paint
        egg cartons cut in half (to hold apples while artists paint
            them)
        brushes
        water container

paper towels
sample apple with decorations — not painted red like a
    real apple

Activity

1.   Distribute materials on table and have one apple at each place.

2.   Begin the group with a discussion of school days (see above). Allow time to reminisce.

3.   Discuss the act of giving an apple to a teacher. Ask: "Have you ever done that?"

4.   Talk about learning as we get older. Ask: "Does all learning stop when we finish school? How are we still learning? What kind of learning are we now doing? For example, are we learning how to get along with others? Are we learning how to propel a wheelchair? Are we learning a new leisure skill?"

5.   Ask each person to think about something s/he would like to learn in the next 6 months.

6.   Using the acrylic paints provided, ask them to decorate their apples to somehow give the impression of what it is they would like to learn. (Have a sample done, so they get the idea that these apples do not have to be red.) An example of this may be, if a person wants to learn how to play cards, s/he can paint cards on the apple. If they want to learn how to get along better with others, they can paint an image of people holding hands. No words at this time.

7.   Use the egg cartons to hold the apples as they paint them, turning the apples on their sides as necessary to cover the entire apple.

8.   When the apples are dry, allow the clients to print significant words on the apples with the fabric paint (you may want to assist here) to further describe their goals.

9.   As the final touches are being put on, discuss the goals for learning they have set up for themselves. Ask: "What might you need to reach your goal? Who do you see as being a teacher of this?"

10.   Allow the apples to dry for 24 hours before allowing them to leave with the clients.

This process combines reminiscence with current events and goal setting.

With lower level clients, have apples pre-painted in red and use the process as a discussion group with you writing the words on the individuals' apples to remind them of their goals. You can also write things they have deemed "the most important things I have learned." Display the apples in a non-eating area or hang them in a way that keeps clients from confusing them for real apples.

Similarly Dissimilar

Size	**4 to 8**
Functioning	**high to medium**
Time	**40-60 minutes**
Purpose	**group dynamics, teamwork, fine and gross motor, abstract thinking**

The beauty and challenge of collage work is often in the unlikely combination of elements. The following project was inspired by a donation received from a seamstress. I received a mind-boggling assortment of patterned material and felt it would be perfect to use with a group. Using fabric allows the client to use materials that are both familiar and non-threatening, and this process further challenges them to work together with other group members in a collaborative effort to achieve a common goal.

I approach this process by stating that they are to work as a team (2 - 4 clients on a team around a table) to complete a fabric collage mural. They are to use the fabric provided and the only rules are

1. They are to apply each piece of fabric to the background so that one piece touches or overlaps another. None of the background fabric should be visible.
2. They cannot use two pieces of the same material right next to each other.
3. They must work as a team, consulting each other as necessary to create a unified piece.

Materials

(for each team of clients)
a large piece of a dark-colored, smooth fabric
approximately 24" x 28"

a wide variety of patterned fabric made of similar
material (I used all-cotton fabric that was donated),
the wilder the patterns the better. Look for fun
Hawaiian shirt fabric and bold color prints as well as
your basic stripes and polka dots!
scissors
white glue
wooden dowel 26" long to hang your final piece from

Preparation

1.   Have each table prepared with the base fabric laid out so
that it is within reach of all group members. Split the
fabric remnants up into piles for distribution to the
teams. Cut remnants in irregular shapes and sizes ahead
of time if your clients have difficulty with scissors.

Activity

1.   Place clients in teams around the tables. Group them
according to abilities in the sense that you have balance.
For example, I placed a woman who was able to stand
up and move around with a group that might have
trouble reaching the center of the fabric. "Mary" could
stand and fill in the center or assist the other team
members.

2.   Begin a discussion of collage. Ask: "Can dissimilar
things be used together to create something aesthetically
pleasing? Is it possible to combine objects that are
different and have them 'work' together?"

3.   Ask them to use the material provided to create a group
collage. Pass out the material so that all can reach it.
Discuss the "rules" for this process as described above.

4.   As they finish the placement of their material, supply glue bottles and instruct or assist them in gluing the fabric down.

5.   As each team finishes, ask the team members to come up with a title for their piece. My group named them "Gone with the Wind" and "Mixed Emotions" because of the mishmash effect of the piece.

6.   Next, begin a discussion of what it was like to work on a project with other members of the group as a team. Ask: "Was it difficult? Why? Is it possible that we are much like the material we work with, that we are all very different people, yet we are able to come together and create?"

7.   Then ask: "If you had to pick a pattern from the material we used that best reflects you, which would it be?"

8.   When the glue has dried, make a hem at the top of the piece and hang it from a dowel. Display it with a title and note about the process used to make it.

The goals for this process are obviously group dynamics, fine and gross motor skills, and abstract thinking. This same process can be used with less verbal or lower level, more confused clients with some variations. Have material precut, incorporate different textures to add a sensory element to it, and focus on color identification, direction following, attention span, and group awareness. This process is both fun for your clients and a good assessment for abstract thinking abilities and to assess their abilities to work with others. The finished product will be wild looking and fun in that sense. It will look best if displayed against a dark or black background.

Clay Doodles

Size	4 to 10
Functioning	any
Time	40-60 minutes
Purpose	fine motor, self-expression

Doodling has been a pastime of human beings probably since cave man days. Wherever there have been sticks and dirt, there have, I imagine, been doodles! Doodling is an art form that is unplanned and at times revealing about our inner thoughts and obsessions. Doodling is a great process to do with a group if it is approached without fear, without forethought, and with a sense of fun.

Doodling in clay provides this activity with a legitimate and permanent surface, giving importance to the task as an art form.

Materials

Laquna self-hardening clay (Laquna is a self-hardening
   clay that requires no kiln or oven baking, if you have
   access to a kiln, regular clay is just as good!)
rolling pin
carving tools (dowels sharpened in a pencil sharpener
   work great)
newspapers
water
sponges
oil-based stain
heavy twine

Preparation

For each group, place the clay on a sheet of newspaper and roll it into a slab 24" x 22" with a thickness of 1". A slab of this size is good for 4 - 5 clients to work around.

Activity

1. Seat clients at the table around the slab, making sure that all of them can reach the center of the slab comfortably.

2. Talk about doodling. Ask: "Are you a doodler? What kinds of things do doodler's doodle?" Talk about it as an art form, an uncensored, fun kind of way for people to clear their minds.

3. Hand out carving tools and instruct them to play in the clay, doodle, scribble, as long as it is unplanned and spontaneous, whatever comes to mind.

4. Allow 15 - 20 minutes to fill the slab with doodles.

5. When complete, smooth rough lines with a damp sponge or finger. Redraw the lines if necessary.

6. Using a butter knife, cut the slab into irregular rectangles like so:

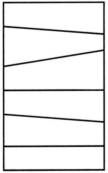

Fig 5.1

7.   Separate the pieces and make holes in the top and bottom corners for later hanging.

8.   Dry slowly, or follow directions for the clay type used.

9.   Finishing: When completely dry, antique slabs by painting over the surface with an oil-based stain. Mayco perfect touch, oil-based stain acrylics are made for antiquing ceramic ware. Rub off with a damp sponge and allow stain to color the doodles and cracks.

10.   Finally, tie together the completed slabs with heavy twine, leaving a space between them of approximately 1/2".

The result you achieve will be somewhat prehistoric or organic looking, uncensored and infused with images and random thoughts from the client's daily lives.

Tiny Bubbles

Size	**4 to 8**
Functioning	**any**
Time	**40-60 minutes**
Purpose	**breathing, reminiscing, sensory stimulation**

What is it about blowing bubbles? Hand any man, woman, or child a jar of bubble solution and a wand and immediately they gleefully fill the room with iridescent bubbles. It seems to remind us all, from any generation, of happier days spent worry and care free. There is also something spontaneous and uncontrollable about bubble blowing that makes it a great challenge to an artist. "How?" you might ask. Well, not only can an artist appreciate the natural beauty of the free-floating bubble, but s/he can also use bubbles as an art medium. Combine food coloring and bubble solution to provide an opportunity to make the brief beauty of the bubble into a lasting artistic expression.

Materials

plastic spoons with various sized holes punched in them (with a single hole punch)
bubble mix (dishwashing liquid, water, sugar)
food coloring
cottage cheese container tops to put the bubble mix in
thin, white, non-textured paper to line the work surface
aprons for participants

Preparation

1. Make bubble mixture following this recipe: 1 cup dishwashing liquid, 1 cup water, 1 tablespoon sugar (to make the bubbles last longer).

2.   Divide the mixture up into many small containers and add 1 - 2 drops of food coloring to the mix.

3.   Cover table surface with plastic tablecloths or newspaper and then with white paper as your art surface.

Activity

1.   As clients come into the art area, hand them an apron and line them up on one side of the table.

2.   Begin a discussion of bubbles. Ask: "Do you remember blowing bubbles as kids? Did your children ever play with bubbles?"

3.   Next, explain that they are about to experience blowing bubbles in a new way. They are going to paint with them!

4.   Explain the procedure of adding food coloring to the bubble mix and ask them to blow bubbles into the air over the paper using the spoons with holes in them as the wands. Enjoy the visual spectacle of colored bubbles in the air as they change colors and land wherever they may.

5.   Assist with the correct blowing technique. (To my surprise some of the clients had difficulty blowing bubbles. Help them blow with the right amount of force to achieve bubbles.)

6.   Sometimes if the bubbles don't blow into the air, the dye may drip onto the paper, let them know that it is all right and is just another part of the image to be.

7.   Rotate colors among participants. When the paper is covered with overlapping bubbles (or people begin to hyperventilate), the image is done.

8.   End the group by discussing what it was like to blow bubbles. No matter what the results of the artwork were,

the clients enjoyed the remembered feeling of being carefree. It just seems to go along with the act of bubble blowing!

I did this group with medium cognitive and physically able clients. Some of my co-workers tried it with various other level clients and were able to achieve similar results, with different amounts of assistance.

I guess tiny bubbles really do make you feel "warm all over."

Three-Dimensional Life Orb

Size	**4 to 8**
Functioning	**high (medium and low with assistance)**
Time	**40-60 minutes**
Purpose	**fine motor skills, sensory stimulation, life review**

Many of us have heard of the creating "Lifelines." Lifelines are done in the image of a historical time line. The reviewer creates a straight line on a piece of paper and then marks locations on the date bar to indicate times when significant things happened. The following process uses this idea, but adds an artist's touch. The paper becomes a spherical ball and the indicators of significance are fabrics and textures that inspire the viewer with an actual "feeling" of the event. This process requires the use of two hands to hold and wrap the ball. Have extra hands available to help this day if some of your clients have difficulty in this area.

Materials

> Styrofoam balls, 6" diameter
> stick pins
> strips of various fabrics and textures approximately 20" long such as: leather, cotton, flowered and patterned fabrics, bright and dark colors, satin, velvet, burlap, yarns, sequins, ribbons, etc.
> scissors

Activity

1. Begin by having all of the items spread out on the table within reach. Precut fabrics to 20" length by 1/2-inch width for easier application to the ball.

2.   Discuss life review. Ask participants to think about stages of their lives where they have grown, changed, or experienced things that are significant to them. Some common answers will be going to school, first date, meeting spouse, getting married, having children, career changes, and death of parents.

3.   Looking at the materials provided, can they find a fabric that could represent by feel or look some of these significant time periods?

            NOTE: Participants can braid or intertwine materials to signify a period when many things happened at once.

4.   Ask them to choose fabric elements, and lay them out on the table in a historical order.

5.   Taking the Styrofoam ball, apply the first fabric piece to the ball by pinning the end of it in one spot and wrapping the material over the ball. Secure the other end with a pin also.

6.   Continue to wrap the ball in the chosen fabrics or yarns in the order they appear in their historical layout. Encouraged participants to overlap and change direction with their fabric application so that all layers can be viewed at some point on the ball.

7.   When all fabrics have been attached to the ball, the client may chose to attach a final piece from which to hang the orb or, instead, leave it as is, so it can be held in the hand.

8.   When all group members are finished, encourage them to share the significance of their fabric choices with the group if they wish. (This discussion can also take place after pieces are laid out in historical order, before placement on the ball.)

9.   Ask: "What is the overall effect of the finished ball? How does it feel to the touch? Does the combination of the fabrics and threads, intertwined and overlapped, make the ball stronger or weaker? When you look at the final image, does it appropriately reflect how you feel about your life history to date?"

10. For members who feel that the orb is too harsh and unsatisfying, ask them how they could change the "feel" of the ball. Invite them to choose another fabric that may represent something they have yet to do, to change the overall weight of the ball.

If you are not comfortable with dealing with life review issues, you can change the theme of the layered ball to a representation of the many layers of their personality. This would inspire a much more lighthearted group, yet still offer the opportunity to deal with issues regarding life review and personal history.

Maps

Size	**4 to 8**
Functioning	**any**
Time	**40-60 minutes**
Purpose	**reminiscing, abstract thinking, fine motor skills**

Have you ever looked at a map in lighting better than the dome light in your car? Maps can be very beautiful, showing texture and color in a unique way used only by mapmakers. There is a sort of artistry about maps that can lend itself to collage work and stimulating discussions on many different levels and degrees of ability. Everyone has a certain familiarity with maps (or at least folding them!) and the use of them in art making is novel and engaging.

Materials

a variety of colored maps from around the U.S. or the world, these can be acquired through donations from your local automobile club or map store as well as being found in all those *National Geographic* magazines you get donated

scissors

black construction paper, 8" x 11"

glue sticks

Activity

1.   Begin the group with a discussion about maps. Ask: "What have your experiences with maps been? What are they used for?" Talk about how interesting it can be to look at maps of places you may never have been. It's sometimes fun to experience and to learn about a

territory in a concrete sense without actually ever going there.

2. Distribute maps on the table. If the maps you get are large, precut them into manageable sizes (8" x 11" or smaller).

3. Ask the participants to look at the different colors on the maps, the textures, and the lines. Encourage them to create a collage with the map itself as their art media.

4. Using scissors or by ripping, create pieces in abstract forms or concrete images, whatever the artist chooses.

5. Glue onto black background. Overlapping is fine.

6. When all are finished, ask them how they used the map as an art tool. Were they able to stop thinking of it as a navigational tool and look at it as more of a color and texture source?

Options

1. With lower level clients, precut the maps into geometric shapes, or let them rip them to create the collage. They might surprise you with their recollections of their map experiences.

2. You may also use the maps to create fantasy trips to different locations. You can cut shapes into them such as boats or kites that may depict some of the things they could do there. Use your imagination as your guide!

Fleeting Images

Size	**4 to 8**
Functioning	**high to medium**
Time	**40-60 minutes**
Purpose	**self-discovery, fine motor skills**

Our lives are full of impermanence. Fleeting images pass through our lives at every moment. Do we take the beauty that surrounds us, for however long it lasts, for granted? The beauty of a sunrise or sunset, of a meteor shower or the brief palette of fall colors in autumn, all fleeting. This group focuses on learning to accept and appreciate a moment of beauty without having to "own" it. It also challenges the artist to create an image for the shear joy of creation, realizing that it is just another brief moment of beauty to appreciate and let go of.

I use colored sand for this project, which you can create by one of two ways. 1. Mix sand and food coloring together to create different shades and colors. Add a bit of water to mix if necessary. Spread the sand on newspaper and let dry. This method gives you a wide variety of possible colors. 2. You can mix dry sand and dry powder tempera paint together to create your media. This method leaves a lovely color "ghost" on the black construction paper work surface and actually gives the artist a hint of the creation after it has been brushed away.

Materials

colored sand in a variety of colors
small shallow bowls
spoons for each color
one sheet of black construction paper per client

Activity

1. Discuss beauty and impermanence. Ask: "What are some examples of fleeting beauty? Do we appreciate the beauty of a sunset less because it is a momentary experience or do we appreciate it *more*?"

2. Pass out the black paper and distribute the colored sand in shallow bowls, a spoon for each color.

   NOTE: never use bowls and spoons in art processes with clients who are confused as they may think there is food involved and eat your materials!

3. Invite the clients to create a beautiful image or design using the colored sand, applying it to the paper using the spoons. Let them know that when they are finished the images will be brushed away.

4. Allow 20 minutes to work.

5. When complete, look at each person's pattern or image. Ask: "Was it difficult to create something beautiful knowing that it would be a fleeting image? Were you able to develop and enjoy the making of the image or design in spite of the final intent? Can beauty be both fleeting and timeless at the same time?"

6. After some discussion, pass around a shallow bucket and ask each person to shake his or her picture off into the bucket. If you used powder tempera to create your colored sand, you'll see a ghost image on the paper. What does that look like? Does it reflect the image of its origin?

If some of your clients have difficulty letting go of their sand painting, you might ask if they have trouble letting go of other things. Ask why they feel they need to keep their work permanently?

You may also want to show pictures of American Indian or Tibetan sand painting as examples of commitment to beauty for the purpose of ritual (specifically a healing ritual).

Most clients come away from this group with a greater appreciation of the joy of creating without the fear of or forethought about "what will happen next."

Sometimes we need to be reminded it's not the destination, but the journey.

The Weight of the World

Size	**4 to 8**
Functioning	**high to medium**
Time	**40-60 minutes**
Purpose	**self-discovery, self-worth, remotivation, fine motor skills, connecting with nature (sensory stimulation)**

Throughout our lives, we accumulate unexpressed feelings, regrets, unachieved dreams, etc. We allow these issues to weigh us down, many times holding us back from accomplishing wonderful things, getting to know wonderful people, or at the very least, from appreciating ourselves. The following process helps us address the need to rid ourselves of the issues and negative thoughts that hold us back and weigh us down.

Materials

medium to large stones in a variety of shapes and colors
    (can be found at the beach, park, or nature areas)
    they should have at least one smooth side
waterproof permanent markers, in a variety of colors
raffia (a papery shredded string available at all craft
    supply stores) or thin twine, cut into 3-foot lengths
a black box big enough for all the rocks

Activity

1.   Ask: "How do you weigh something down?" Talk about the feeling of being weighed down. What kinds of feelings or circumstances "weigh us down?" Some answers may be worry, pain, financial hardship,

heartbreak, greed, and envy. Allow discussion of some specific times when each person has felt weighed down.

2.   Ask each person to think of several things or times they have felt weighed down. Keep those thoughts at the front of their minds.

3.   Place the stones on the table within each persons reach. Instruct the clients to choose 3 to 5 stones each. One for each incident they have thought of.

4.   Place the markers on the table and ask the clients to indicate the issues they have thought of, in words or images, by drawing them on the rocks.

5.   Once complete, pass out lengths of twine or raffia and instruct the clients to wrap the string around the rock, going around it many times, as if tying up a package. Let them know they are "binding" these negative thoughts and occurrences so that they may be disposed of.

6.   Assist with tying off the strings and cut any remaining string off. Participants may completely cover their stone, indicating a real desire to end the power of the things that weigh heavily upon them.

7.   When all are complete, ask each member if s/he is ready to get rid of the things that bind him/her.

8.   Ask members of the group to place their stones into the black box.

9.   Let them know that by placing their worries into the box, they have taken them out of their world and have locked them into a place where they will no longer hold them back or hold them down.

10. End the group by talking about feeling unburdened. A mind unhampered by worry has more time to grow, be creative, and to love.

This group is designed to be both therapeutic and non-threatening. It allows the artist to address issues of independence in a private way, and still gain strength and support from the group.

Flying Free

Size	**4 to 8**
Functioning	**high to medium**
Time	**40-60 minutes**
Purpose	**reminiscing, abstract thinking, self-worth**

The following process deals with an issue that is important to clients of a health care facility on either a long-term or short-term basis. Freedom. So many things are decided for them, out of their control, that they are often left with the feeling of being in a prison, unable to determine things for themselves. This process uses the image of a paper airplane as a concrete way of turning our need to fly, to feel free, into a reality in at least some small way.

Materials

drawing paper, 12" x 9"
craypas, crayons, or markers
paper clips

Activity

1.   Discuss the phrase; "free as a bird." Ask: "What does that mean to you? What would it be like to soar over the earth? How would that feel? Or to fly in a hot air balloon or an airplane? Do you think it would be a peaceful feeling?"

2.   On the paper provided, ask them to create an image that would reflect that feeling, either in form or color. Ask them to fill the entire surface of the paper if possible.

3.   Once all are complete, look at each image. Ask: "What does that image represent?"

4.   Afterwards, ask them all to turn over their pictures, (picture side down) and take them through the step-by-step process of folding their paper into an airplane. As you go, see if they can guess what it is they are making. Assist clients with correct folding if necessary.

5.   When folds are complete add a paper clip to the middle bottom fold to hold it all together.

6.   Let their images soar.

With an older group, a lot of reminiscing was going on about making paper airplanes or kites as kids. Doing the test flight of their planes was a great way to re-experience the carefree feeling they had as youths. Younger groups focus more on how they will soar in the future. Although this process requires the ability to think abstractly for the image making, you can implement this group with lower level clients. Have them decorate the paper and, after you fold the airplanes, feel the freedom of flight as they sail the airplanes. It's great if you can do your test flights in a big room to enhance the feeling of freedom. It is surprising how such a simple fold of paper can bring a smile to a face, and a feeling of freedom that should not be forgotten.

The Shell

Size	**4 to 12**
Functioning	**high**
Time	**40-60 minutes**
Purpose	**self-discovery, reminiscing, self-worth, fine motor skills**

The image of the egg conjures up many thoughts... more than just "breakfast!"

The egg shape is considered a universal symbol for wholeness and rebirth. Conversely, in nature, the size, color, and shape of the egg usually indicate something about what's to be found inside. There are fragile-shelled eggs, and eggs that are buried by their mothers for protection. If we were to think about our own "hatching" and growth over the years, what kind of egg (form of shelter and protection) would we have come from? Would we be a fragile-shelled egg, frail and uncertain, or would we be bold, colorful, announcing our arrival to be a thing of consequence.

This process looks at the symbolism of our development by asking high-level participants to take ownership of the egg image, and to impose upon the wooden egg provided something of themselves. Through color and line they can develop an eggshell that illustrates something of their journey, as individual as their own growing process.

Materials

wooden eggs, available through many craft supply stores or through Sax Arts and Crafts catalog (800-558-6696)[1]

---

[1] If your eggs come with wooden cup stands, as they do from Sax, spray paint those gold ahead of time to be used to display the finished product.

stabilizing trays[2]
acrylic paints
small paintbrushes
water
gold paint or spray paint

Activity

1.   Begin the group with a discussion of the egg. Ask: "What is the purpose of an egg or an eggshell? What symbolic meanings can you think of that could pertain to the egg?"

2.   Distribute stabilizing trays as needed, wooden eggs, and paints to each participant. Ask them to imagine themselves as hatched from an eggshell like a bird might be. What kind of shell would it be? (See introduction). Ask them to take 20 minutes and create an eggshell that would represent something of themselves, their journey, and their growth.

3.   Encourage the use of color and line to illustrate moods and feelings regarding their journey.

4.   Encourage the use of a main color as background on the egg, to be painted on first in a wash type manner. For example, paint the whole egg with a light blue paint wash first before further development. A wash is a watery flowage of color onto a surface.

---

[2] Stabilizing Trays: Many people find it difficult to paint a three-dimensional item because of the need to hold it while working. To help individuals with paralysis due to stroke or other types of problems, create a stabilizing tray using old cottage cheese containers or even old egg crates. Fill the container with dry plaster or sand. Cover loosely with plastic wrap or paper towels. The artist may place the egg at any angle in the sand or plaster and work on one area at a time, allowing the paints to dry before changing positions. This device allows the artist independence and comfort during an otherwise challenging process.

5.   As eggs are finished, set them in the wooden egg stands that have been sprayed or painted gold ahead of time. State that since their eggs house the spirit of their journey, the images of their growth, they should be treated with respect and honor.

6.   When all are complete, look at each egg creation and discuss images.

The images and conversations that are brought up during this process might surprise you. You may even find some of your eggs have cracks painted onto them. Some of your clients may feel as though they are damaged (cracked) but remind them that all eggs have to crack at some point in order for the treasure inside to be born.

Genie in the Bottle

Size	4 to 8
Functioning	high to medium
Time	40-60 minutes
Purpose	remotivation, self-worth

The myth of the genie has crossed many cultures and ages to become a universally known story. You find a magic genie in a lamp or vessel; you set it free by rubbing the vessel; and the genie is so grateful for his freedom that he grants you three wishes. What those wishes are tells of the master's greed, or ignorance, or big heart and consideration. Those wishes are oh, so revealing, and have been the fodder for many a dinnertime conversation.

The following process offers the group participants the opportunity to not only question themselves about what their three wishes would be, but also offers them a creative opportunity to become familiar with their own genie.

Materials

clean, 20 oz. plastic soda bottles with caps or corks to fit
colored metallic or silky ribbons
iridescent papers
colored tissue paper or colored cellophane
Modge Podge ™ mix (available at art supply stores or
    use glue and water mixture)
sponge brushes to apply the mixture
scissors

Activity

1.   Begin the group by discussing the story of the genie. Ask them to imagine themselves finding a genie. Ask:

          "What would it look like? What would the vessel look like?"

2.   Using the materials supplied: tissue, iridescent papers, and Modge Podge, ask them to create their own genie vessel. They may cut shapes from the papers and apply them with the Modge Podge or just tear irregular pieces and apply.

3.   Begin the covering process by spreading a thin layer of the glue on the bottle and then pressing on the paper or tissue. Cover tissue with glue and continue the layering process, always spreading a layer of the Modge Podge or glue over the last layer of papers.

4.   When the vessels are covered to their satisfaction, allow them to dry. Tie colorful ribbons around the lip of the container to dress it up a little more and seal up your genie with the cap of the soda bottle, or buy corks that will fit the opening of the bottle.

5.   As the bottles dry, discuss the three wishes they may have. Ask: "What do your wishes say about you? How can you achieve your dreams without a genie?"

6.   As you end the group, have the group think of themselves as genies. Ask: "Can you make someone else's wishes come true? Can you make your own wishes come true?"

    Members of this group leave the session considering the possibility of their own abilities to make things happen, and to free the genies inside themselves. A truly magical experience.

Great Balloon Creations

Size	**4 to 8**
Functioning	**high to medium (low with modifications)**
Time	**40-60 minutes**
Purpose	**self-expression, fine motor skills**

Throughout the country, people may get the chance to visit and view the grandeur of the great hot air balloon races or exhibitions, where national groups share the beauty of color and pattern, comical or commercially decorated balloons, with the general community. Anyone who has ever seen this spectacle will tell you of the vibrant colors and intricate patterns. Each balloonist appears to try to outdo the others.

With this in mind, invite your moderate to high level clients to let loose their creativity on the very challenging media of the helium balloon.

Materials

permanent markers in various colors (metallic markers are available and provide visually exciting results)

balloons, various sizes and shapes

helium source

ribbon

tape

photos of hot air balloons (available from your local library, just ask!)

Styrofoam cups and scissors for adaptive equipment needs

clear plastic garbage bag

Activity

1.   Have a variety of balloons filled with helium and tied with a ribbon. Keep them under a clear plastic garbage bag so they don't float away.

2.   Show pictures of the hot air balloons and discuss the creativity of color and design. Invite your group members to be unofficial hot air balloon designers.

3.   Have clients select a balloon to decorate from the ones provided.

4.   Take the ribbon that is tied to the balloon and tape it onto the table so the balloon is touching the table surface.[3]

5.   Have the artists to create designs on their balloons using the permanent markers.

6.   Remind artists to work all the way around the balloon.

7.   Participants can use several balloons to create a sculpture. Attach the balloons together with tape or ribbon to create a more complicated form.

8.   When completed, allow the balloons to float higher over the table. Look at each person's designs and discuss the colors and shapes. What other ideas did they have that they were unable to create?

9.   Clients may take their balloons home with them as a decoration and to remind them of the process.

---

[3] Two hands are needed to work on the balloon in this fashion. If you have people with poor motor control, cut a hole in the bottom of a Styrofoam cup and pull the ribbon through it until the balloon "sits" in the top of the cup. Tape the ribbon securely to the table. This will help steady the balloon, but additional assistance from you may be needed.

Options

1.   With lower level clients, use stickers to decorate the balloon, common "dot" stickers you can find around the office are good for design creation with little effort, cost, or frustration.

This group offers a fun new way to create art, with little preparation or difficulty. It is good to have some volunteers handy to lend a hand to those who have difficulty working on a moving object.

Use of acrylic paints is also good here, as long as so much is not applied that the balloon cannot lift off.

Gauge the level of your clients, and try to ensure that the process is fun and not a frustration to them. A little more prep time from you can help guarantee success for them.

Going Buggy

Size	**4 to 12**
Functioning	**medium to high (low with optional activity)**
Time	**40-60 minutes**
Purpose	**overcoming fears, discovery, creativity**

Bugs. Our initial reaction to the generalized "Bug" word is "Yucko! Hand me a rolled up newspaper and I'll take care of it." However, upon closer inspection, the insect world is full of intricate patterns and, yes, beauty. Up in the North Woods of Wisconsin, I have discovered a whole world of insect beauty, colorful and complex.

Besides the discovery of, and appreciation for, the arachnid as a species of beauty, there's something about studying them as art that removes that "eek!" mentality and helps us overcome our fears. That's what the following process is all about. Overcoming fears by studying the things that frighten us.

Materials

large color photos of a variety of insects or reptiles, (found easily in all those *National Geographic* magazines you get donated, or at the library)
crayons or pastels
black construction paper 8" x 11"
tape
white construction paper for viewfinders

Preparation

1. 　　　　Cut construction paper into 6" x 6" viewfinders with a 2½" x 2½" square cut from the middle.

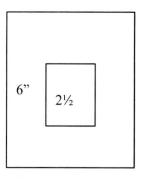

Fig 2.3

2. You might want to isolate the image of the bug by cutting it out and gluing it to a dark background so that the artist is not tempted to use the background as their design inspiration.

Activity

1. Begin with a discussion about insects. Ask: "How do you feel about bugs? Which ones are you afraid of? Why?"

2. Put photos onto the tables; ask clients to take a photo that is most repulsive to them.

3. Can they find anything good or attractive about their bug?

4. Distribute viewfinders; ask them to move the viewfinder over the image of the insect. Look for beauty, patterns, or designs.

5. Once a pleasing image is located, tape down the viewfinder and lay out the paper and pastels. Ask them to replicate the image. Ask them to enlarge the view as if the image were under a microscope.

6.   Look at the results. Discuss their experiences in reference to the following philosophies: "Appreciate beauty wherever you find it," or "Befriend your enemy."

Options

1.   Begin the group with the viewfinders hiding the image of the bug, only allowing the artist to see the pattern. After a discussion of the beauty, reveal the entire picture. Are they surprised? Repulsed?

2.   Line draw some detailed images of insects from pictures. Ask your clients to fill in the outline with outlandish and imaginative colors to make them seem more appealing. (Lower level)

End the group with a conversation about facing our fears, or at least understanding them.

This group was done with medium to high-level cognitive and physical functioning clients. You can use the general idea in other ways with different level clients.

Creator

Size	**4 to 8**
Functioning	**high to medium**
Time	**40-60 minutes**
Purpose	**self-worth, group dynamics, abstract thinking**

If you were able to design your own little piece of the world, what would it be like? Would it be a cityscape, filled with towering high rises, or would it be a rainforest, a desert? Would your world have human beings on it? Would it be hot, cold, filled with living things, or desolate?

These are the questions I asked a group of medium to high-level seniors. The following process is a great creative, easy, and challenging process that stimulates discussion and a sense of control. Asking people to create a new environment challenges them to think in new ways, and establishes a sense of fun and "I can do no wrong."

Materials

blank puzzle sheets in the shape of a circle, available
from Compoz-a-Puzzle (800) 343-5887
magic markers
masking tape
cardboard frame to hold the puzzle in place (optional)

Activity

1. Begin the group with a discussion about designing your own world. Ask members to think creatively. Let them know that they can change our world to what they want their own world to be. Talk about changing colors of things, e.g., sky could be green, water red. The whole planet could be rocks, or furry, or water…whatever they

can conceive. Ask members to think about what they like best of this world and what they like least.

2. Place the circle blank puzzles in front of each member, place some masking tape on the back to help stick it to the table so it doesn't move around a lot while they work. (Better yet, because the tape could hurt the back of the puzzle, cut a frame out of plain cardboard with a center hole the size and shape of the puzzle and tape the frame to the table.)

3. Using the markers, allow them to create an image of what their world would look like.

4. When the new "planet" is complete (encourage them to fill in all the white spaces), ask them to come up with a name for the new world and perhaps write it along the bottom curve of the piece.

5. Look at the worlds created and discuss what each world would be like, and why the artist decided to create it in such a manner.

6. When complete, challenge them to take their puzzle apart and mix up the pieces. Exchange puzzles with other members of the group to solve.

Options

1. Another way to do this process is to use one puzzle, giving each person 1 or 2 pieces to decorate with their own rendition of their world. Putting the puzzle together then, blending each other's ideas, becomes a conversation starter. Ask: "How can these different environments thrive together on one planet? How do our different ideas join to create an unusual and exciting new world?"

2. Creating a group world like this is a great way to introduce new members to the rest of the group, and

helps alleviate the stress of trying to cover an entire circle with one's sometimes-limited ideas.

Overall, this process should encourage fun and imagination. The use of a puzzle blank instead of just a piece of circular paper encourages a game sense instead of a heavy, serious group process.

Either way you do it, *The Creator* process should be a stimulating and imagination-challenging process for all involved.

Building Blocks

Size	**4 to 8**
Functioning	**high**
Time	**two or three 40-60 minute sessions**
Purpose	**reminiscing, self-discovery, fine motor**

People always talk about how a successful business or marriage, or any newborn endeavor, needs a strong foundation to build upon. They talk about how a good relationship or education are good building blocks for a wonderful life or career. It is with this in mind that we ask a group of high-level participants to look at their lives, from childhood to the present, as a series of building blocks. Looking back upon our lives and seeing how one decision leads into the next, can be very eye opening. It helps us to see patterns of behavior, as well as progression in wisdom.

Materials

wooden blocks, approximately 4" x 4" (can be bought at craft supply stores), 7 blocks for each participant
spray paints in a variety of colors
acrylic paints
brushes
3-dimensional paints like Scribblers™ or Renkly™ in metallic or pearlized colors
black permanent markers
water buckets

Preparation

Spray blocks in a variety of solid colors so that artists do not have to "prepare the canvas" prior to decorating it. Make sure you have all possible "emotion" colors represented such as black, red, yellow, white, etc. Have metallic colors available also for those "golden memories."

Activity

1. Begin the group with a discussion of "building blocks" as described above. Ask each participant to think about the 7 most significant decisions or events in his/her life from birth to the present. Some of these events may bring up sad or angry feelings, some may be happy, all should be represented if the artist feels they are significant and have helped to shape the person s/he is today.

    Participants may want to write these events down for later reference, as this may be a 2 - 3 group process.

2. Have clients choose 7 blocks from the prepared blocks provided. They should choose specific colors for the specific events that they will be representing.

3. Starting with their first significant event, their first building block, ask the artists to use shape and color to indicate the nature and emotion of the event. They should carry design over five sides of the block and place their initials or personal "mark" on the bottom so that the blocks are easily identifiable.

4. Continue work on blocks over group meetings as necessary.

5. When all of the blocks are done and dry, ask participants if they would like to share some of the stories behind each event. This will most likely happen naturally as people are working on their blocks if the group is cohesive and comfortable. If they choose not to share their stories, let them know that the group members respect their privacy. Let everyone get a chance,

however, to see the images on everyone's blocks if possible.

6.   Lastly, ask the clients to stack the events in order, as they would conceive the "building blocks" of their lives thus far, being built. Do their blocks rest upon one another; are they built in a tower, or laid out like a map? Ask: "Do you feel that your life has had a direction? Who or what drives you to continue? (For those who tower) Do you feel you are moving upward? (For those who laid their blocks down in a line) Do you feel that your road has been tiresome, or just very clear?"

If possible, take another week for this process to create a bag or container to hold the blocks. You can purchase papier-mâché boxes at craft stores or use covered shoe or package boxes. Make sure that there is enough room in the box for future blocks to represent memories in the making.

Painting by Candle Light

Size	**4 to 8**
Functioning	**high to medium**
Time	**40-60 minutes**
Purpose	**self-discovery, group dynamics, abstract thinking**

For most of us, finding images in unstructured markings has been a challenge to our imaginations since childhood. Finding animal shapes in the clouds, deciphering ink blots or paint splatters, allows the artist to stretch his/her creativity in a way that is both spontaneous and revealing all at the same time. By using a candle's flame to lightly singe watercolor paper, you can create a smoky, ghostly image that can be explored in many ways. Because of the obvious safety risks, you should singe the papers before the group begins and offer your clients a wide range of starting images. Using the method described below, try to create some markings that may suggest different levels of complexity, so that no client needs to struggle with the task.

Materials

watercolor paper, 4" x 6" sheets (prepared as stated below)
black permanent markers
watercolor paints
brushes
water containers
candle

Preparation

1.   Light a candle. Move the paper over the flame quickly. You should achieve a brownish, smoky image on the

paper. Cross your singe marks; vary their shapes and sizes on the paper. Do not make them too complex. Prepare enough so that each member of the group can complete two images. The use of smaller paper is suggested so that the image doesn't get lost on a larger sheet of white paper.

Activity

1.	To begin the group, discuss the challenge of image finding. Talk about the need to stretch the imagination and about the ways we do image finding spontaneously (looking at clouds, finding patterns in leaves, etc.). Explain that the challenge for this group is to use the marks left by a candle flame as the source for their inspiration.

2.	Allow the clients to choose a pre-smoked sheet of watercolor paper. Encourage clients who have more difficulty with abstract imaging to work with simpler designs.

3.	Discuss ideas for each individual image. Let peers assist peers with suggestions if necessary.

4.	Distribute markers. Ask the clients to outline or elaborate on the image they see.

5.	Distribute paints, brushes, and water. Allow 20 minutes total to elaborate on the design as they see fit.

6.	When all are complete, show each person's completed image. Ask: "Was it difficult to create an image out of thin air? Did you see any other images in your starter smudge?"

If using candle flame is not right for you, use bits of charcoal to create the smudges, set with a spray fixative, and proceed with the rest of the process.

Charm Wands

Size	**4 to 8**
Functioning	**high (medium with assistance)**
Time	**40-60 minutes**
Purpose	**self-discovery, fine motor skills**

Wands have been a symbol for magical wonder for decades. We have seen them depicted in fairy tales and fables and have always associated them with something special.

"Charm wands" were traditionally glass tubes filled with seeds and hung over doorways. The story goes that if bad spirits came by while you were at rest, they would be distracted by the wand and would stop to count the seeds, thereby being caught on the wand. Later, they could be wiped off to rid the house of bad spirits.

On that inspiration I went looking for some special supplies and gave my clients the opportunity to create a little magic themselves.

Materials

hollow plastic tubes approximately 14" long, and 3/8" in diameter, one per client

small corks to fit in the ends of the tubes (I got mine from a science and surplus store)

small beads

glitter

miscellaneous small shiny things

masking tape

rubber cement

small funnels

narrow gold ribbon

small shallow plastic cups

Preparation

1. Pour small beads and glitter into smaller bowls or cups so that client's can see the materials clearly.

2. Rubber cement a cork in one end of the plastic tubes.

Activity

1. Have supplies distributed on the table.

2. Discuss the history of wands in general and charm wands in particular. Ask: "What kind of magical powers can you remember wands having? Who used wands?" Distribute the plastic tubes with one cork cemented into the bottom of the tube.

3. Instruct the clients to make their own charm wands, to be used not necessarily to chase away bad spirits, but to rid ourselves of negative thoughts and feelings. Invite them to create their wand with as many materials and colors as they choose.

    Note: Some helpful hints on how to fill your wands may help avoid frustration from shaky hands: One way to fill your wand with beads is to put the beads in the palm of your hand, then kind of shovel them into the wand. Another helpful method to fill your wands is to use a small funnel, taped with masking tape to the end of the tube and to simply fill the funnel with glitter and beads and shake down.

4. As the wands are being finished, apply some rubber cement to the cork, place it in the open end of the wand, and seal. Finish the wand with some gold ribbon tied at the top.

5. When all are complete, ask each client to show his charm wand to the others. Ask: "What kind of magical power would you like your wand to have?" Some

answers I got were "to cure the common cold" or "to lift the darkness." One client I have actually turned her wand into a timeline of her life, explaining the meanings of the different strata of colors.

Really there are no limits on the kind of magic or meaning the creator could establish with his/her wand. At the very least, the wand can remind each of us that there is a bit of magic in all of us, and maybe all we have to do is believe.

Pandora's Box

Size	**4 to 8**
Functioning	**high**
Time	**40-60 minutes**
Purpose	**connectedness, life review, remotivation**

The story of Pandora's box has been a familiar Greek myth to many of us. Roughly, the story is that Pandora was given a box by one of the gods for safekeeping. She was told not to open the box. She did. When she opened the box, all the "troubles" flew out and entered the world. By the time she was able to replace the cover, the only thing left in the box was hope. That is why, the story goes, that despite all the troubles in the world, there is still hope.

The following process reflects on this story and asks the participants to create their own boxes, and their own images of "troubles" and "hope."

Materials

poster board prepared as described below, or plain
cardboard boxes
markers
crayons or craypas
pictures from magazines appropriate for project
rubber cement
scissors
markers

Preparation

1. Create your own boxes. Use poster board and cut it following the template below:

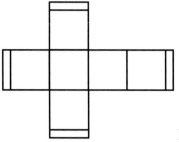

Fig 5.2

2.   Fold at lines. Glue at the tabs to close after the boxes are decorated.

3.   By doing this you can allow the clients to work on the inside and the outside of the box in a flat and easily accessible position. If you are unable to create your own boxes, use pre-formed boxes, spray paint them a neutral color, and proceed with the process.

Activity

1.   Have boxes available on covered tables and discuss the story of "Pandora's Box."

2.   Ask your clients to think about their worries. Create images of their worries on the outside of the box using paints or collage pictures and words. If you want to detach the clients from the project a little, ask them to create images of the world's worries, not necessarily their personal images.

3.   When done, ask them about the things in their life that give them hope. Ask: "How do you keep your hope alive? (Or how do we see hope in the world?)" Create an image of hope on the other side (or inside) of the box.

4.   Put the boxes together with the hopeful images on the inside.

5.   When done, discuss their images. Some of your clients may find this process disturbing; they may have

difficulty finding hopeful images. This is a good opportunity to allow them to express their feelings among friends. Allow other group members to share their ideas on how to maintain hope and how to have a more "hopeful" attitude.

6.   To end the group, remind the clients to try to cast out their troubles, to put them away from themselves sometimes and to reach into the hope that lives within them. "Despite all the world's troubles, there is still hope."

Zen Gardens

Size	**4 to 8**
Functioning	**high to medium**
Time	**40-60 minutes**
Purpose	**connectedness, group dynamics,**
	abstract thinking, fine motor skills

Table-top Zen gardens, in general terms, are shallow sand boxes where the owner or Zen gardener creates simple patterns with a small "rake" device. Most of the time you see them with 2 or 3 rounded stones as accents that the sand designs are created around. The purpose of the Zen garden is to allow the creator a meditative experience where the slow development of patterns results in a calming and restful frame of mind.

In the following process, the art of the Zen or sand garden is used with high to medium level clients to provide that same restful, contemplative experience in a world that may often seem chaotic, noisy, and out of control.

Materials

shallow box tops similar to the kind you get for shirts
plastic forks
feathers
rocks of various sizes with rounded surfaces
sand to fill each box top 2/3 full
soft, melodic music
sample of Zen garden

Activity

1.   Begin the group by displaying a sample Zen garden in the center of the worktable. Have soft music playing in the background.

2.   Discuss the Zen garden as in the introduction of this process.

3.   Distribute box tops and sand. You can allow each person to pour a measured amount of sand in his or her own box or have it done ahead of time.

4.   Distribute the tools for the garden. Place a plastic fork and feather at each person's place. Allow them to choose from the round stones, 2 or 3 rocks apiece.

5.   Encourage everyone to play around with the different patterns they can make in the sand. Can they think of any other tools they could use?

6.   Now, encourage a quiet time of about 10 minutes where each person will listen to the music, and create a pattern in his/her garden using both sand and stones. Clients can easily change their design by wiping their hand over the sand until they are pleased with the effect they get.

7.   If people finish before the 10 minutes are up, they may sit quietly until the group is finished.

8.   When all are done, turn down the music and talk about the feelings they had while creating their garden. Ask: "Do you feel more restful? Did your minds clear in a meditative way or did your day-to-day worries invade your 'gardening' time?"

9.   Discuss the difference between creating a Zen garden and playing in a sand box.

End the process with a comment on whether or not the participants found value in creating a moment of calmness in their day. Ask if they would like to work on their gardens again. Before leaving the group, smooth out the sample garden and ask each member to place a stone from his or her garden into the group garden. As group leader, rake a pattern around the rocks to tie the members together. If practical, keep the garden in the room for a few sessions, inviting a different member each week to reconfigure the sand. The group's Zen garden will serve as a concrete reminder of the comfort and security that being part of the group can be.

Chapter Six

Presentation and Purchasing

The importance of presentation of the artwork created during your groups should not be underestimated. It is the finishing touch that communicates to your group that you respect their endeavors and that their work has merit not only for its process of creation but also for its aesthetic power.

This does not mean everything has to be put under glass. Placing a matte around paintings or drawings and hanging them on a wall in your day room or facility corridors is sufficient. Ideally, budget permitting, purchase a Velcro display wall or board that can hold artwork of various shapes and dimensions.

Creating a note about the process of the creation and the names of the artists (with their permission only!) gives the participants pride in being part of a creative group and helps explain the significance of the work.

Finding a glass display cabinet or other protected area to place larger creations, such as the life orbs or the apples for the teacher, is the best. If you can't assure the security of work like this, keep it displayed in protected areas like an activity room or art room. Always let your artists choose whether to display their work, keep their work, or dispose of it. Privacy and confidentiality are a big concern when working with art therapy processes. You want the client to feel open to express himself or herself during a group without fear of reprisal or embarrassment. The choice to share their thoughts in the group as well as the choice to share their art with the rest of the facility is theirs alone. They are the owners of their creation and you must respect that.

Many of the collage plans suggest using the finished project for sensory stimulation tools. The colors of materials, the texture of fabrics or woods can be utilized by other therapists to help assess cognitive abilities or to test orientation.

Any of the artwork displayed in your facility will be starters for discussions between staff and clients or between clients and family. Generally, the participants of your groups will feel that they are a part of a select group and show pride in their accomplishments. I had one client that would sit near the artwork during the day so that he could explain the process and the thoughts behind the creation. He shared his value of the group with others in hopes of fostering more understanding and support for the art programs at my center.

Selling artwork is sometimes a question. It is very flattering to the individual if his/her artwork is admired to the point of purchase. I generally pass along the interest to the clients and let them decide if they want to part with their creations. I always suggest to the buyers that they send a personal thank you card to the clients to let them know that their work is appreciated and valued.

Finding time to display artwork properly is difficult. Your supervisor may not think it is a good use of your time either, and you need to educate him or her that it is part of the process. Feeling pride in one's accomplishments can heal self-worth issues and provide a client with the feeling that s/he is more and greater than his/her disability. A person can reach farther by looking into himself/herself and expressing that self outward. Sometimes having a paintbrush in hand helps.

Art Supply Resources

The following stores carry art supplies that may be used with the activities in this book and for all of your other art projects. Companies sometimes change the products they carry, so you may have to hunt a little for some of the more unusual items. All of the items were available the day this book went to press.

Compoz-A-Puzzle, Inc.
One Robert Lane, Glen Head, NY 11545
Phone: (800) 343-5887
Fax: (516) 759-1102
Web: http://www.compozapuzzle.com

Dick Blick Art Materials
PO Box 1267, Galesburg, IL 61402-1267
Web: http://www.dickblick.com
Phone: (800) 828-4548
International: (309) 343-6181
Fax: (800) 621-8293
Customer Service: (800) 723-2787
Product Info: (800) 933-2542
E-mail: info@dickblick.com

JuneBox.com, Inc.
W6316 Design Drive, Greenville, WI 54942
Phone: (800) 513-2465
Fax: (800) 513-2467
E-mail: info@junebox.com

Misterart.com – online shopping

Nasco
901 Janesville Ave., Fort Atkinson, WI 53538
Phone: (800) 558-9595
Fax: (920) 563-8296
E-mail: info@eNASCO.com
Web:www.eNASCO.com

Nasco — Modesto
4825 Stoddard Rd., Modesto, CA 95356
Phone: (209) 545-1600
Fax: (209) 545-1669
     E-mail: modesto@eNASCO.com

Potpourri Artist's Supply, Inc.
Suite E, 6663 El Cajon Blvd., San Diego, CA 92115
Telephone: (619) 697-7366
Order Desk: (619) 697-7717
Toll-free: 1-888-697-7717
Web: http://www.potpourri-art.com

Rex Art
2263 SW 37 Avenue, Miami, FL 33145
(305) 445-1413 Fax (305) 445-1412
(800) REX-ART2 ((800) 739-2782)

Sax Arts and Crafts
PO Box 510710, New Berlin, WI 53151
Phone: (800) 558-6696

Glossary

3-D fabric paint usually dispenses from a squeeze bottle with a narrow tip; this is a specially created fabric paint that leaves a raised trail of paint when applied. Great for writing on fabric or outlining.

body paint a specially made, FDA-approved paint for application to the skin. Colors usually last several days but can be removed with alcohol.

brayers small, hard rubber rolling pin type applicators for paints or printing inks. Comes in many sizes with a handle. Allows for thin, even coat application for printing techniques.

camel hair paintbrushes a soft, economy paintbrush made generally for watercolor painting.

chalk pigmented artists chalks come in small sticks. Used dry for drawing or sketching, they are powdery and blend easily. Used wet they appear more vibrant in color and are less smudgy.

charcoal pencil a drawing pencil, with varying degrees of hardness; allows an artist to sketch with charcoal, with the convenience and cleanliness of a pencil-style coating.

colored pencil pigmented, softer lead pencil used for drawing or sketching.

core spacers small squares of foam core board, used to raise objects off of the construction or drawing surface.

crayons (wax) pigmented wax with a paper wrapping, used for drawing or wax resist. Offers a grainy surface coverage.

Craypas a brand of oil pastels; these drawing sticks offer a creamy, blendable alternative to the wax crayon.

face paint a specially designed paint that can be washed off with soap and water. Usually found on a stick and applied with a brush. Similar to clown paint.

hand over hand technique refers to a therapist assisting a client by lightly guiding the client's hand in the process of a task.

kiddie tray paints an economical version of watercolor paints; usually seen sold as a set of nine or twelve colors; paints are weak in color and grainy when applied.

linear the use of a line; having only one dimension.

markers water based, non-toxic pigmented inks in a pencil type form, can be applied to most papers easily, but with little ability to blend.
- wide tip – larger tip for maximum coverage.
- fine point – narrow tipped for writing or fine work.
- washable markers are available, otherwise inks are permanent.

matte a textured cardboard-like frame with a 2" to 3" margin, used to frame artwork. Can be cut with a matte cutter or bought in common sizes pre-cut.

Modge Podge a brand of glazing liquid with a glue-like base. Can be used to seal projects or to create a shine over a surface. Spreadable with a paintbrush.

mount to affix artwork to a wall for display. Example: a picture can be mounted to a wall.

oil pastel an oil-based, pigmented coloring stick; gives a solid, creamy effect to drawings.

paintbrush tips the part of the brush used for painting; different tips are used for different reasons:
Squares – good for creating hard lines in paintings.
Rounds – nice for a softer application of paint; usually used with watercolors.
Angled – used in acrylic painting to give hard lines or textured effects.

palette any non-porous surface that holds artist's paints; usually made of Masonite board, porcelain, or plastic.

palette knife a wide, tapered metal knife with a bend, used to scrape paint from a palette, blend colors, and apply acrylic and oil paints to a canvas.

paper different papers are appropriate for specific projects:
- watercolor paper — textured, high cotton content paper that accepts water-based paints, especially watercolor paint, offering flowing coverage while the texture is visible.
- student grade watercolor — less forgiving with less cotton fiber present; this paper is fine for beginners but cannot be overworked without paper saturation and tears.
- finger-paint paper — a wax-coated paper with a slick surface that allows heavy paint application and can be used with printing techniques. Does not absorb the color as other papers do and tends to wrinkle and get wavy as paint dries.
- animal prints or printed papers — great for use in collage work, usually thin and not appropriate for paint. Can be torn or cut and adhered to other surfaces with a thin coat of glue or tape.
- poster board — a heavier paper, with a variety of available colors; good for backing artwork for display or for art construction projects. Can be used with markers or crayons, but does not hold paint well.
- railroad board — a much heavier paperboard, difficult to cut, but can be used much like matte board. Usually smooth

surfaced, works nicely for mosaic projects and with people with fine motor skill problems as it has dimension and weight.

Renkly brand of non-toxic, three-dimensional paint.

Scribblers brand of non-toxic, three-dimensional paint commonly found at craft supply stores.

sponge brushes a paintbrush with a sponge head in place of the usual hair or bristle tip. Used for application of acrylic paints and watercolor washes.

stabilizing tray adaptive equipment that holds a piece of artwork while an artist works. Can be made from common household products such as Styrofoam cups, egg cartons, or sand bags, depending on the shape and size of the object being worked on.

student grade watercolor paper see paper.

synthetic paintbrush used for oil or acrylic paints, the bristles of the brush are made of synthetic fibers, which allows for clean, controlled application of heavier bodied paints.

watercolor paper see paper.

Index

About the Author

Diane Fausek-Steinbach has been facilitating art therapy groups with long-term care, rehabilitation, and general population clients over the last 14 years. She has authored *The Practical Guide to Art Therapy Groups* (Fausek, Haworth Press, 1997) and writes a monthly column for Creative Forecasting Inc. on art therapy processes with seniors.

Currently, she is the Director of Senior Center Programming for Interfaith Older Adult Programs, a non-profit organization with programming that enhances the quality of life for older adults in the Milwaukee area.